TRANSFERENCE

*Its Structure and Function
in Psychoanalytic Therapy*

TRANSFERENCE

Its Structure and Function in Psychoanalytic Therapy

BENJAMIN WOLSTEIN, Ph.D.

Introduction

CLARA THOMPSON, M.D.

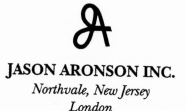

JASON ARONSON INC.
Northvale, New Jersey
London

THE MASTER WORK SERIES

First softcover edition 1995

Library of Congress Cataloging-in-Publication Data

Wolstein, Benjamin.
    Transference : its structure and function in psychoanalytic
therapy / by Benjamin Wolstein
        p. cm.
    Originally published : New York , Grune & Stratton, 1964.
    Includes bibliographical references and index.
    ISBN 1-56821-626-2 (alk. paper)
    1. Transference (Psychology). 2. Psychoanalysis 3. Psychodynamic
psychotherapy. I. Title
RC489.T73W65   1995
616.89' 17—dc20   95-16993

Manufactured in the United States of America. Jason Aronson Inc. offers books and cassettes. For information and catalog write to Jason Aronson Inc., 230 Livingston Street, Northvale, New Jersey 07647.

TO IRMA

Contents

Introduction

DURING THE LAST TWENTY-FIVE YEARS, there have been many outstanding changes in the theory and technique of classical psychoanalysis. Prior to 1925, the goal of analytic therapy was the removal of the infantile amnesia. It was thought that neurotic difficulties developed because significant memories of early childhood had become repressed and "forgotten." The theoretical assumption was that, if these memories could be recalled to consciousness, the source of the neurotic disturbance would be removed and the patient would be well. The method used to facilitate the recall was named *free association*. The patient would lie on a couch and faithfully report whatever came into his mind. Since he had come to a physician for help with his problems, it was to be expected that the things uppermost in his mind at the time would be thoughts relating in some way to his complaints.

As Dr. Wolstein has shown clearly in this book, the method had a goal similar to that achieved by hypnosis, as it was practiced in the latter part of the 19th century. The patients did, in fact, recall painful and traumatic experiences relating to their difficulties, and, often, the recall was therapeutically effective. However, Freud soon discovered that the method did not always work smoothly. There would occur periods when nothing was in the patient's mind, or when the patient would talk about trivial and unimportant things.

At first Freud coped with this difficulty by authoritative suggestions, e.g., "When I press my hand on your head, something will occur to you." This often worked. Presently it became apparent that the most frequent cause of blocking was thoughts relating to the analyst. The patient hesitated to say something of which he was ashamed for fear the analyst would think less of him, or he had a critical or unfriendly thought about the analyst, or, especially in the case of women, there were erotic phantasies about the analyst.

In short, the patient feared disapproval or punishment from the analyst, and behaved like a frightened or naughty child. Freud concluded that the attitude must be a revival of early childhood reactions to parents, and thus transference was discovered. Since this is the chief topic of this book, I do not wish to discuss transference in any detail, but merely to point out that there are two ways of using transference therapeutically. One may use the patient's exaggerated positive attitude to increase one's influence with him. That is, if you are the all wise loving father, whatever you say will have great weight with the patient. This attitude was undoubtedly fostered in patients in the early years, although, at the same time, Freud made strenuous efforts to keep suggestion out of the picture. Still the fact that nothing should be done to weaken or destroy the authority of the analyst must often have encouraged an attitude of blind obedience in the analysand. As Dr. Wolstein has documented, this type of therapeutic use of the transference was the standard procedure before the nineteen-twenties.

The second way in which the transference can be used therapeutically grows out of the fact that by observing the attitudes of the patient, as expressed towards the therapist, both people can obtain insight into how the patient relates to people in general, especially how he relates to authority figures. This insight will help clarify how he himself contributes to his difficulties in living. In using the transference in this way, it becomes the central interest of the analysis. The shift from using it in the first way, i.e., to reinforce the authoritarian power of the analyst, to using it in the second way began in the nineteen twenties.

Several other important changes also began at about this time, and were related to the new attitude towards transference. The emphasis on the recall of the past as the chief goal of therapy began to be questioned, and there was a trend towards greater emphasis on understanding the analyst-patient relationship. By 1930, Ferenczi was saying it was therapeutically useful for the analyst to admit when he had made a mistake—that this actually helped the patient test reality. That is, he questioned the usefulness of doing nothing to destroy the authority of the analyst.

Harry Stack Sullivan began about this time talking about the analytic situation as an interpersonal process in which the personality of the analyst also figures. The defensive functions of the ego began to be studied, and more and more the recall of the past has come to be seen as important only to the extent that it helps the patient understand his present life situation. However, not until about ten years ago did analysts in general accept the importance of acknowledging the ways in which their own personalities were involved in the therapeutic procedure.

In the last few years, there are an increasing number of studies of the role in therapy of the countertransference, i.e., the emotions and attitudes of the analyst towards the patient. So analysis has progressed from its authoritarian origin in hypnosis to a democratic present.

Through all these changes, Dr. Wolstein has followed the changing concepts of transference with scholarly precision. Dr. Wolstein is eminently qualified for the research he has undertaken. He is trained in three disciplines, philosophy, clinical psychology and psychoanalysis. He has always had great interest in the development of scientific theory. I believe this book is an important contribution to the understanding of the theory of analytic therapy and it gives me great pleasure to participate in its production.

CLARA THOMPSON, M.D.

Executive Director, W. A. White Institute of
Psychiatry, Psychoanalysis and Psychology
March 1954

Preface to the Second Edition

WRITTEN TWELVE years ago and published two years later, this study is now being reprinted with major additions and minor corrections. Psychoanalytic inquiry, as conceived in this study, sustains itself without the direct support of either biology or sociology, and requires no more than a self-consistent metapsychology for its formulation and procedure. Further studies, done since then, extend this perspective into wider areas of clinical theory and practice.[1] Certain notions that first appeared in *Transference*, however, are still useful: unconscious aspects of current experience, observable sequences of anxiety and distortion in the therapeutic present, relativities of transference and countertransference, dynamic continuities of conscious and unconscious processes—of impulse, intelligence, attitude—in every transaction of patient and analyst, and therapeutic analyses of the human psyche

---

[1] See B. Wolstein, *Countertransference*, New York: 1959, and *Freedom to Experience*, New York: 1964. Also, see "Some Comments on the Field of Psychotherapeutic Inquiry," *American Journal of Psychotherapy*, VII (1953), pp. 503–514; "On a Neglected Aspect of Freud's Psychoanalytic Procedures," in *Proceedings of the 7th International Congress of the History of Science*. Paris: Hermann & Cie, 1953; "The Analysis of Transference as an Interpersonal Process," *American Journal of Psychotherapy*, VIII (1954), pp. 667–678; "Psychoanalysis as the Study of Transference," *Acta Psychotherapeutica, Psychosomatica et Orthopaedagogica*, III (1955), pp. 735–742; "Transference and Immediate Experience," *American Journal of Psychotherapy*, XI (1957), pp. 277–292; "Mysticism and Psychoanalysis," in *Progress in Clinical Psychology*. New York: Grune & Stratton, 1958; "The Unconscious Present in Psychoanalytic Therapy," *American Journal of Psychotherapy*, XIII (1959), pp. 283–297; "Transference: Historical Roots and Current Concepts in Psychoanalytic Theory and Therapy," *Psychiatry*, XXIII (1960), pp. 159–171; "Existential Analysis in Search of a Therapy," *American Journal of Psychotherapy*, XV (1961), pp. 382–394; "The Limitations of Mysticism in Psychoanalysis," *Psychologia*, V (1962), pp. 140–145; "On the Psychological Absurdity of Existential Analysis," *Psychoanalysis and the Psychoanalytic Review*, XLIX (1962), pp. 117–124; *Irrational Despair*. New York: Free Press of Glencoe, 1962; Review: "The Scope of Psychoanalysis: 1921-1961, The Selected Papers of Franz Alexander," *American Journal of Orthopsychiatry*, XXXIV (1964), pp. 598–602; and "The Unity of Psychoanalytic Therapy," in *Proceedings of the 6th International Congress of Psychotherapy*. London: 1964.

as systematic inquiry, above all, but as distinct from various speculations about its metapsychology. Two special appendices are written for this second edition, the first recording a historical chapter that was omitted in 1954 so as to explore more carefully the unexplored roots of Freud's analysis of transference in late nineteenth-century hypnocathartic therapy, the second bringing up to date other related metapsychological and procedural issues. Corrected, also, are the original page-proofs to meet valuable suggestions of several reviewers, especially Dr. Silvano Arieti's, *American Journal of Psychotherapy*, IX (1955), pp. 109–110; Dr. Paula Heimann's, *International Journal of Psychoanalysis*, XXXVII (1956), pp. 491–493; and Dr. Jerome Singer's, *Journal of Abnormal and Social Psychology*, L (1955), pp. 410–411. To

those colleagues, students and friends, as well, who have offered their often challenging yet always welcome criticisms, I am deeply indebted; I now thank them all, fully and gratefully. With equal pleasure, again, I thank Mr. Jules Altman for generously and thoughtfully helping to get this new edition ready for publication.

                                                              B. W.

Faculty, W. A. White Institute of Psychiatry,
Psychoanalysis and Psychology; Clinical
Professor of Psychology, Adelphi
University, New York City,
April, 1964

Preface to the First Edition

THIS STUDY is not a systematic codification of our current knowledge of transference phenomena. It is not a conceptual analysis of the interrelationship of the various theories of analytic therapy. Nor is it a handbook of therapeutic technique. It is the result of confronting Freud's last theory of transference with current theory and practice. I have attempted to set forth a new perspective in which to consider the analysis of transference as a therapeutic instrument. When Freud discarded the hypnotic and pressure procedures in favor of the technique of free association, he failed to expand the fabric of analytic therapy beyond the aims of recovering lost memories and overcoming resistance to their recall. In this study, the psychoanalytic theory of transference is taken out of the framework of hypnotic goals in which he had left it, and an operational definition of transference distortions is constructed and supported.

The psychoanalytic tradition in which this study may be placed has been identified with the work of Fromm, Fromm-Reichmann, Horney, the Riochs, Sullivan and Thompson. They have all contributed to the reevaluation of Freud's biological frame of reference and to the reconstruction of his therapeutic procedures—both of which have made way for the cultural and interpersonal framework for understanding psychological disorder. And the philosophic tradition in which it may be placed is that of James, Dewey and Mead, who have in our day reasserted man's ability to study the structure of process without developing a platonistic underpinning to explain its timeless essence. In both his life and work, William James epitomized the quest for personal freedom from preconceived absolutes. John Dewey worked out the logical and social analyses through which the need for crystal-clear certainty might be surrendered. And together with George Herbert Mead, they are responsible for the philosophy of experience in which the belief in social intelligence supplanted blind reliance on hardened dogma.

The analysis of transference distortions is really at the heart of analytic therapy. The occurrence of distortions in the transference relationship is not taken to be qualitatively different from their occurrence under ostensibly non-therapeutic conditions. The analyst does not have to be or do anything out of the ordinary range of everyday experience for them to occur, while their formation and communication is affected by what he is and does. This, in a word, is the point of view which will be worked out here. It has grown in part out of my own clinical experience with transference distortions; in part out of the theoretic and therapeutic conceptions now associated with the William Alanson White Institute of Psychiatry, Psychoanalysis and Psychology; and in part out of the shortcomings of Freud's essentially hypnotic approach to transference which became increasingly clear on the basis of both the clinical experience and the interpersonal conceptions.

I am happy that Dr. Thompson has introduced this study on such a crucial subject. Her early contribution during the thirties now stands among the landmarks pointing in the direction which the development of transference analysis eventually was to take. She was among the first to distinguish valid transference experiences from transference distortions and see the centrality of this distinction among the current factors in successful analytic therapy. And my indebtedness to her is somewhat more personal, for she has taught me the significance of following through on the subtle intricacies of transference distortions.

I am also indebted to her and to Drs. Ralph M. Crowley and Edward S. Tauber for reading various drafts of the manuscript and making many excellent suggestions and constructive criticisms about its organization and content.

My thanks are due the following publishers for the privilege of quoting passages from their publications: Basic Books, Inc., New York: quotations from *Sex in Psychoanalysis* and *Further Contributions to the Theory and Technique of Psychoanalysis* by Sandor Ferenczi; Hermitage House, Inc., New York: quotations from the lectures of H. S. Sullivan in *The Contributions of Harry Stack Sullivan,* edited by Patrick Mullahy, by special permission of the W. A. White Psychiatric Foundation, Washington, D.C.; The Hogarth Press, Ltd., London: quotations from *Collected Papers* by Sigmund Freud; Houghton Mifflin Company, New York: quotations from *Counseling and Psychotherapy* by Carl Rogers; Nervous and Mental Disease Monographs, New York: quotations from *Studies in Hysteria* by Joseph Breuer and Sigmund Freud; W. W. Norton & Company, New York: quotations from *The Psychoanalytic Theory of Neurosis* by Otto Fenichel, *An Outline of Psychoanalysis* and *New Introductory Lectures on Psychoanalysis* by Sigmund Freud and *New Ways in Psychoanalysis* by Karen Horney; University of Chicago Press, Chicago: quotations from *Principles of Intensive Psychotherapy* by Frieda Fromm-Reichmann; and the W. A. White Psychiatric Foundation, Washington, D.C.: quotations from "Countertransference and Anxiety," *Psychiatry,* XV (1952), pp. 231–243 by Mabel Blake Cohen.

I also want to express my gratitude to Mr. Jules Altman who made many critical suggestions, read page-proofs and compiled the very thorough index, and to Mrs. Nora Holland who saw the typescript through its various stages and attended to numerous other details. And my appreciation of my wife's cooperation is only partly reflected in the dedication of this work to her.

B. W.

Clinical Psychologist, Low Cost Psychoanalytic Service,
W. A. White Institute of Psychiatry, Psychoanalysis and
Psychology; Psychologist, Therapeutic Services, Post-
Graduate Center for Psychotherapy; New York City,
February 1954

chapter one

The Major Shift

OF THE THREE ASPECTS of Freud's work—diagnosis, treatment and theory—the decision about his greatest accomplishment now rests with what it holds for current psychotherapeutic technique, for psychoanalysis stands or falls as a method of treatment. It was Freud of course who laid the groundwork of psychoanalysis as a therapeutic instrument, and this was his genius. To take note of this fact without reference to the extraordinary courage he showed in publishing his findings as he saw them would necessarily be incomplete. We must pay tribute to Freud's fearlessness as a scientist even though the results of recent investigation have ruled out equal tribute to his theoretic formulations. That he himself began to doubt the efficacy of analytic therapy around the twenties should not blind us to his fundamental contribution. He had opened up a new scientific frontier in which he was followed by many outstanding workers in Europe and America, the remarkable thing being that he had built better than he knew.

By now it is clear that his observations in the analytic situation have far more lasting value than either his diagnostic categories or his theoretical framework. Since psychoanalysis is essentially a therapeutic study of interpersonal processes, it follows that his early diagnostic formulations can have little contemporary claim to acceptance—no more than his later ideas about characterology which were based on libidinal development. The descriptive diagnoses are not essential because therapeutic communications are not radically affected by them. The general psychoanalytic technique is similar, though not identical, in practically all cases, and modifications in approach are introduced in response to changes in the ongoing therapeutic situation. And his character typology has extremely limited utility because it suffers from a one-dimensional bias, and fails explicitly to encom-

pass effects of social structure and of cultural values on the formation and communication of interpersonal attitudes.*

Freud's profound observations of the workings of the human
mind are cornerstones of a scientifically grounded psychoanalytic
psychology. But the groundwork of a science does not constitute
the science. During the last fifty years, psychoanalysis has undergone many basic revisions and modifications, and if Freud were
granted the opportunity to review the results of his handiwork,
he probably would not be able to recognize them. In fact, some
outstanding workers in the field have not only refused to be considered neo-Freudians; they have even avoided identifying their
psychological therapies with Freud at all. One need not look far
afield to learn why these changes were made. There were many
questions implicit in his point of view which he had left unanswered, and many new ones have arisen which transcend it. In all
fairness, it must be pointed out that definitive conclusions have
not as yet been reached about them. The large-scale system of
psychoanalytic psychology designed to deal with all possible contingencies has not been constructed, and it is not altogether fruitful to speculate whether or not it ever will be constructed. A
short-range piecemeal approach to concepts which specify recurrent observations and their operational definitions is replacing
the omniscient quest for the grand scheme.

The Freudian views about the nature of man, the origins of his
problems and the therapeutic procedures to resolve them, actually combine into a systematic philosophy of life. This philosophy is deeply embedded in the intellectual traditions of the eight-
eenth and early nineteenth centuries. Now it is not necessary to
subscribe to the assumptions of Kant or Hegel or Schopenhauer
in order to practice psychoanalytic therapy. It can be .practiced
with at least equal efficacy even if one finds the philosophic perspectives of other thinkers more congenial. Indeed the German
idealist tradition, with the convergence of Kant's formalism, Hegel's dialectic and Schopenhauer's pessimism in the latter half of
the nineteenth century, found itself in a number of social and
scientific dilemmas. Even though Freud tried to avoid their im-

* See *Appendix B* (1964), pp. 234–238, for comments on the interpersonal
perspective.

plications by adopting a physiological base for his psychology, his methodology landed him in many insoluble contradictions which permeate the entire body of his work.

The major defects of late nineteenth-century metaphysics and scientific method have already been worked through in current inquiries in the philosophy of science. Those philosophic positions have already been thoroughly overhauled and reconstructed. And there is no cogent reason why the recognition of these defects in the foundations of psychoanalysis does not require a corresponding reconstruction in both metapsychology and therapy.

It has been an unfortunate historical circumstance that philosophy and psychoanalysis have developed along parallel lines which converged on few and scattered occasions. Freud often noted the remark that there is more in heaven and earth than philosophers ever dreamed of, and he could do this with a certain equanimity because it was supported by a host of astute clinical observations which had no place in the established philosophies of human nature. Extreme wariness developed quite early in the history of psychoanalysis about the possible constrictions of philosophy, and this was undoubtedly reinforced by the hostile reception which Freud's great discoveries were initially accorded. This wall between philosophy and psychoanalysis has had detrimental effects in both fields, but not equally so. Philosophers have not only begun to dream about the importance of unconscious processes in their theories of ethics and human nature; they are even beginning to reformulate some of their basic conceptions. Psychoanalysis has not fared quite as well. For it is quite evident that there is more in recent philosophy of science than Freud ever dreamed of, and contemporary psychoanalysis has generally failed to take account of its implications. I am referring to the operational point of view which has been applied very fruitfully in physics, biology, sociology, animal psychology and the logic of science.[1]

[1] For sample writings in these disciplines, see P. W. Bridgman, *The Logic of Modern Physics,* New York: 1927; J. W. Woodger, *Biological Principles,* London: 1929; R. K. Merton, *Social Theory and Social Structure,* Glencoe, Ill.: 1949; B. F. Skinner, *The Behavior of Organisms,* New York: 1938; and

Now it is of course true that twentieth-century psychology stands on Freud's shoulders. But it is more important to see why contemporary psychoanalysis had to climb onto his shoulders: obviously his profound insights brought new perspectives into view for both theory and therapy. Some may take the attitude from the very outset that the limitations of classical theory are necessary for the continued application of its insights, but only an obscurantist would blindly hold that a new approach is foredoomed to failure because of the entrenched dicta of past practice. And it would be a curious blindness which overlooked the revolutionary applications of the operational point of view in these other sciences. Meyer, Cameron and Sullivan have already made fresh starts in the reformulation of psychoanalytic theory in accordance with its leading principles and techniques with varying degrees of success.[2] The need for the reexamination of logic and methods is being felt in the most exact of the empirical sciences, and psychoanalysis, a comparative newcomer in the family of sciences, cannot do better than to follow this lead in the measure that its techniques and subject matter permit. To reevaluate methods and results on the basis of operationism cannot but be beneficial, for this new point of view affects the basic postulates of all human knowledge.

What is operational analysis? A definition is considered to be operational when it is defined in terms of the activities by which it is derived, and when such derivation and definition can be specified by means of checking operations. What a definition or term means is to be found by observing what is done with it

---

J. Dewey, *Logic: The Theory of Inquiry*, New York: 1938. For an integrated discussion of this point of view against the background of the "subject-object" theory of knowledge, see J. Dewey and A. F. Bentley, *Knowing and the Known*, Boston: 1949.

[2] Both A. Meyer (*The Commonsense Psychiatry of Dr. Adolf Meyer*, edited by A. Lief, New York: 1948) and N. Cameron (*The Psychology of Behavior Disorders*, New York: 1947) have sought to systematize their concepts from this new point of view, but their contributions have not been geared to interpersonal processes in which therapist and patient engage to the same extent as H. S. Sullivan's (*Conceptions of Modern Psychiatry*, Washington, D.C.: 1947). See, however, Cameron's recent turning to Freud's biological metapsychology (*Personality Development and Psychopathology*, Boston: 1963).

rather than noting what is theorized about it. This approach is geared to the factual observations openly and undogmatically, and it is especially sensitive to their dependence on the actual operations by which they are secured. These empirical operations are obviously not identical with the definitions they require. To hold that a procedure is identical with its definition or explanation is a confusion which is at once useless and obstructive to any sort of knowledge. For whatever else is called for in the formulation of a definition, there must be the operation of the process of generalization. With the appearance of new data, we are compelled to decide whether to refine our definition and include them or whether to construct a new one to characterize them.

All observations and definitions in any subject matter have a place somewhere along a continuum. At one end are those with a maximum of empirical support, while those with little or no relation to factual evidence are at the other. It is obvious where many of the metapsychological theories fall, but it is also obvious that there is much room for clarity and refinement in the myriad of psychoanalytic observations and definitions. Briefly put, psychoanalysis is concerned with the therapeutic treatment of psychological disorders, with the processes involved in participant observation, with the logical and interpretative steps which intervene between observations, definitions and their systematization into an organized body of knowledge.[3] Thus it qualifies as an empirical science if its observations and definitions are specific and unambiguous in meaning; if they briefly describe and explain the psychological processes to which they refer; if they are consistent with one another and with our knowledge in other fields; and if they are fruitful in their application and lead to the discovery of new facts.

Having stated the operational conception of knowledge in brief, I hesitate to continue without noting the very real and very great difficulties it encounters in a field like psychoanalysis where unconscious processes are so significant and where the per-

[3] See B. F. Skinner, "The Operational Analysis of Psychological Terms," *Psychological Review*, LII (1945), p. 270.

sonality differences among analysts make a specific procedure operationally valid for one but not for another. Furthermore, psychoanalytic theory and therapy constitute a very young and growing field. Practitioners who adhere to the various schools report positive results irrespective of diverging tenets and conflicting frames of reference. The metapsychological beliefs and assumptions do not seem to be as important in the actual therapeutic process as the interactions through which analyst and patient integrate interpersonal situations. Taking this cue a bit further, the science of psychoanalysis will probably grow as more attention is given to the therapeutic art of influencing clinically manifest difficulties favorably. In the long run, this will probably turn out to be more useful than the defensive clarification of orthodoxies which do not emerge directly in the therapeutic process.

This question of focussing upon and clarifying the procedures of analytic therapy is more intricate and much more complex than it is in physics or even in experimental or animal psychology. For example, the role of language and communication, the congealing effects of conventional mores and institutionalized practices, the repression of some attitudes and the uncritical transfer of others from one situation to another—such factors are hardly relevant in the study of animal behavior and where molecular entities of physical matter are being investigated their relevance is decidedly secondary. The proper study of man is still man, and though we may get fruitful cues from other sciences, we cannot overlook the significant characteristics which are peculiar to interpersonal attitudes and deviations in the social behavior of men. And these characteristics will be worked out more fully later in this essay.

As developed in the exact sciences, operational analysis requires certain refinements which are very difficult to secure in the human situation. Thus its stipulated requirement to maintain constant and identifiable conditions during an experiment has been a major obstacle in the way of its direct importation into psychoanalysis. In physical experimentation and to a lesser extent in animal experimentation, it is possible, while the independent variables are being controlled, to follow through the changes of the dependent variable if and only if all of the other conditions are kept constant and invariable. This type of procedure produces reliable knowledge because it makes it possible to observe and ascertain concomitant variations in the behaviors of two isolable factors, the independent and dependent variables. If, however, the initial conditions cannot be experimentally controlled, as in the case of analytic therapy, it becomes impossible to decide whether the intervention of other unidentified variables has not affected the behavior of the dependent variables isolated for observation. Clearly, the operational point of view has to be modified in this and other respects so as to adapt it to the statement of psychoanalytic procedures as they actually go on in practice. For if its requirements of establishing certain conditions as constant and invariable during an experiment were literally and rigidly adhered to, its utility in psychodynamic research and therapy would be nullified.

Since the analyst cannot possibly hope to institute and control the initial conditions under which he takes a patient for analysis, he can only work with the facts as he finds them, follow their leads and respond to them in order that the patient discover in himself new and favorable conditions of change. And in view of this latter goal, he does not have and does not permit himself the liberty to experiment with troubled human beings in the manner of laboratory science, mathematical logic or chess. For the analyst is enjoined by the nature of his goals from carrying on psychological research which will interfere with presumably assured human satisfactions. This basic difference veers the study of interpersonal processes away from the quest for universal laws of human nature, assuming such laws exist or can be constructed, and it requires full concentration on experienced difficulties and the concrete details of their occurrence.

Indeed, so far as the immediate concerns of analytic therapy go, the significance of interpersonal processes to which we respond is conditioned by our responses to them. What they are prior to clinical experience is often difficult to say and impossible to ascertain, for they cannot be significant—cannot, literally, bear signs—before they are encountered and experienced; they are what they are and do what they do, and nothing more can be said about them. The assignment of meaning, however, may emerge only from experiencing them. The meaning of experienced processes involves more than the specification of the immediate experiences involved, for the experience of processes is a necessary as distinguished from a sufficient condition of significance. Even if one is out of sympathy with this point of view and insists on separating what a definition means from the way in which it procures meaning, he may still consider the proposal that all definitions are at least implicitly operational in that they are bound by the observations which condition their formation.

Nothing more need be asserted about the nature of interpersonal processes than accumulated knowledge permits, and nothing final can be asserted until, if it were humanly possible, all of the operational possibilities have been executed. If human behavior should at any future date fail to exemplify traits attributed to human nature, then psychoanalysis may call upon this proviso—that its definitions refer to operations of inquiry and treatment: when interpersonal processes change, operations of inquiry and treatment change, and of course our knowledge of these processes changes. Fallible human beings select and organize facts into hypotheses which are ineluctably limited; some are better, others worse; some succeed, others fail. For hypotheses are verifiable or unverifiable to the extent that selections of fact are adequate for the purpose to which they are put. Whatever else human nature may be, it is at least those traits which can be experienced, described and known. If the field of psychopathology is defined in terms of observable behaviors, and communication is one characteristic mode of human behavior, then the definition of the psyche may be postponed so far as scientific inquiry is concerned. And if, moreover, the key to neurosis is transference distortion, its meaning need not be analyzed in relation to the psychic stuff of human nature.

Perhaps the chief virtue of operational analysis is its freedom from outmoded conceptions. Universal laws which had been traditionally defined in terms of properties, forces or instincts maintained a status antecedent to—and, hence, independent of—the modes of investigation by which they were established; behavioral events had essential natures, fixed forces or instinctual bases governing their definition. As long as science clung to this medieval doctrine, its conceptual scheme was bound to be subjected to revolutionary changes at frequent intervals; for as new knowledge was obtained, the frame of reference had to be refashioned accordingly, and the metatheory had to be adjusted to the verifiable inferences, the fundamental source and ultimate justification of scientific postulation.[4] Operationism is essentially an insistence that scientific observations cannot be defined in terms of antecedently defined properties, that traits of knowledge in one field are not to be imposed uncritically on the pursuit of knowledge in another field, and that there is no need to decide in advance of observation and definition on the metatheoretical characteristics of all future results of inquiry. Thus it seeks to eliminate violent and recurring changes in the philosophic account of various scientific subject matters.

Known facts are given a metatheoretical status only after the empirical investigations have been carried out, and metatheory may ascribe only a relative, tentative and unfinished status to its results; all empirical knowledge has this provisional character. As a result, philosophic speculation about scientific findings has been placed on firmer grounds, and the conception of science in relation to philosophical speculation about it has undergone a salutary change. This drastic change in viewpoint may be epitomized by the reconstruction of the "subject-object" theory of knowledge which had been utilized in nineteenth-century varieties of ideal-

---

[4] "Metatheory" is used here to refer to the type of intellectual analysis which goes beyond the actual workings of any organized science. This term is introduced to take account of the metapsychology which Freud created as well as traditional metaphysics which may be traced to Plato and Aristotle in Western thought.

ism, rationalism and empiricism. In these traditions, the theory of knowledge was triadic: it postulated a realm of objective materials, empirical operations involving them and the definitions resulting from operations. So long as this dualism of the knower and the known was considered valid, the objective materials maintained a position independent of the observer. But the critical reconstruction began to take hold in America at the turn of the century, and so this dualism began to break down.[5] It soon became clear that the "objects" of knowledge were inextricably related to knowing "subjects," and the knowledge that resulted was dependent to a large extent on how the knower carried on his procedures of observation. Thus the object of knowledge no longer enjoyed a privileged place which could be isolated from the perspective and procedures of the observer. The theory of knowledge is consequently construed as dyadic, and its major concerns now involve observations and definitions. What we do with natural materials are starting points of knowledge, and these activities of the observer get at the crucial data out of which hypotheses are formulated and leading definitions are arrived at. The so-called objects of knowledge are not the starting points of inquiry; they are denotable conclusions of it. The knowledge of

5 In psychological theory, James had attacked the mechanistic conception of consciousness in his famous chapter on the stream of thought in Volume I of his *Principles of Psychology*, New York: 1890, and Dewey's epochal paper on the dynamic reinterpretation of the "complete act" appeared six years later under the title, "The Reflex Arc Concept in Psychology," *Psychological Review*, III (1896). On the scientific side, Dewey published his *Studies in Logical Theory*, Chicago: 1903, in which he set forth the basic ideas of his situational theory of knowledge; A. W. Moore, an outstanding defender of this point of view, later collected a significant, though unfortunately neglected, series of essays entitled *Pragmatism and Its Critics*, Chicago: 1910; and G. H. Mead had already begun to develop his social theory of consciousness which was published in mature form in *Mind, Self and Society*, Chicago: 1934. And of course there was C. S. Peirce who was working at his new doctrine of "pragmatism" from 1871 onwards; the following three papers provide a good summary of his views: "What Pragmatism is," *Monist*, XV (1905), "The Issue of Pragmatism," *Monist*, XV (1905) and "Prolegomena to an Apology for Pragmaticism," *Monist*, XVI (1906).

objects is thus a process of which objects of knowledge are products.

When these products and conclusions of inquiry are themselves taken as facts to be inquired into, their metatheoretical traits emerge. When we proceed from the results of specific scientific investigations to the most general traits of human existence, that is to metatheory, one important reservation is made. The results of metatheoretical inquiries may deter free inquiry in the future, and so their intrusions into the selection and organization of factual evidence are kept at a minimum. The validity of the metatheoretical enterprise is not denied from an operational point of view, but a caveat is entered that it do its abstract job of analysis and integration and set forth the metatheoretical status of some segment of observed behavior only after we know what it is and only after we know what it can do.[6] What happens to scientific facts after they have been reliably observed and carefully defined is a philosophic concern which does not deflect from the integrity of the procedures by which they were originally defined and organized. Succinctly stated, philosophy of science is concerned with the implications of scientific findings for a systematic view of the world and man's place in it, while specific sciences follow through the development of operational definitions from their starting point in observations and back to them.

Operational analysis may be criticized or rejected because of habitual and emotional attachments to medieval doctrines, but such attachments are not to be confused with its limitations. It has already demonstrated its ability to resolve old problems in new and more precise ways. The factors instigating the search for universal laws in psychoanalysis are historically grounded in conceptions of science which have been superseded. Contemporary analytic theory could not avoid arriving at an impasse because of

[6] See J. H. Randall, Jr., "Dualism in Metaphysics and Practical Philosophy," in *Essays in Honor of John Dewey*, New York: 1929, for discussion of the utilitarian purposes to which various types of metatheories are put; also, see his recent *Nature and Historical Experience*, New York: 1958.

the marked duality between highly abstract and even confusing
metapsychological laws and specific and concrete interpersonal
difficulties. With the needs for a workable technique and a consistent and applicable terminology as pressing as they are, we
may seriously consider operational analysis as a possible har-
binger of a really scientific psychoanalytic therapy. The other
alternative—that constructs and procedures be grounded in nineteenth-century views of science and human nature—is scarcely a
preferable one.

The close scrutiny of Freud's views has in fact been going on
in this country for the last twenty-five years. One outstanding
result has been the realization that no single-factor theory of personality can be established on the basis of purely psychological
findings. The quest for the fundamental laws of instinctual psychology no longer yields fruitful points of departure. Fortunately,
the tendency to make sweeping generalizations and defend absolute statements is becoming increasingly curbed in psychoanalytic formulations. The reason for this newly found wisdom will
become more apparent if we inspect the pattern of analysis in
Freud's concept of sexuality. In an ambiguously wider sense of
the term, sexuality was considered the single basic determinant
of human behavior, and it was also used to explain social thought
and action. Interpersonal disturbances were seen as symptomatic
representations of the patient's sexual life, while the converse
possibility—that his sexual activities be taken as symptomatic of
disturbances in interpersonal relations—was ruled out *ab initio*.
This method, often referred to as reductionism, did not tolerate
a multiple or pluralistic conception of conditioning factors; it
found its chief support and rationale in a monistic point of view.
Yet any such view of the source of interpersonal and social processes is in fact reversing the actualities involved. By divorcing the
external side of human activities from their internal side, interpersonal processes were isolated from ongoing social experience.
They were translated into sexual metaphors with an "electric
current" conception of libidinal energy whose movements, dis-
placements and permutations were taken to account for events

in both modes of experience. These sexual metaphors were then read into the so-called instinctual structure of human nature, and they were finally used, as a sort of anti-climax, to explain the very things from which they were derived and adapted in the first place. Consequently, when psychoanalytic findings were conceptualized in this way, social science became a magnificent tautology.

This methodological approach was introduced quite early in the history of psychoanalysis. It has never been altered; it has, to my knowledge, only been elaborated. Rather enlightening is a cursory comparison of Freud's idea of this pattern of analysis in 1905 with his posthumously published discussion of it in 1948: changes in viewpoint and method are difficult to discern.[7] But this separation of interpersonal processes from environing social conditions severely limits the possibilities of socializing imaginative vision and understanding which often point beyond those conditions. It reduces interpersonal psychology to social behavior or defends the existence of an intrapsychic residue beyond the social category; and either way, the analysis of problematic conditions in living is placed in an insoluble predicament.

One of the best ways to illustrate such shortcomings is to inspect Freud's use of the Oedipus myth. It provides an instructive example of how a residue of intrapsychic processes can be denied intimate contact with environing conditions. As a definition of his field of inquiry, the Oedipus complex actually produced a mythological description of the familial situation. Aside from any question about the reliability of his interpretation, there is something very questionable about the general symbolic utility of this ancient myth. If we remember that Freud acknowledged quite openly and candidly that his instinct theory was a mythology,[8] our quandary about his profound concern with the Oedipus story

---

[7] See S. Freud, "My Views on the Part Played by Sexuality in the Aetiology of the Neuroses," *Collected Papers,* Volume I, London: 1924, pp. 272–283 and compare it with Chapter II of *An Outline of Psychoanalysis,* New York: 1948.

[8] S. Freud, *New Introductory Lectures on Psychoanalysis,* London: 1933, p. 131.

only increases. For it lifted the study of specific difficulties as experienced in living out of the historical situation in which they were lived and experienced. It cut a broad swath across the continuities of experience and severed these difficulties from the cultural aims and institutional practices which entered into their formation and persistence. It brought about a very contradictory state of affairs: mythology had lifted Freud's enterprise out of the context that gave it rise and meaning, while his theoretic notions about childhood and feminine psychology were, at the same time, firmly rooted in the social and cultural traditions of his era. And his insistence on the metapsychological necessity of this myth becomes even more puzzling because it runs counter to an astute clinical empiricism which yielded such great discoveries as resistance and transference.

Freud obviously knew and took account of more about his times than he was willing to admit into his psychoanalytic theories. Why he did not openly introduce cultural considerations would be incomprehensible if we overlooked the scientific atmosphere in which he lived. His desire to secure universal and inviolable principles was a product of his era; it was deeply rooted in the nineteenth-century philosophy of nature and human nature. For example, in one place, he depicted his *homo psychologicus* as a separate encapsulation; the psyche was only open at the bottom, at the no man's land where it supposedly joins the soma, but it lacked any open and direct channels of communication with others in its environment.[9] His views on human nature and psychoanalysis were nurtured by the scientific climate of opinion in which he worked and thought. They are no longer considered valid or useful. Recent developments in social characterology and the interpersonal conception of feelings and attitudes reflect this generally changed perspective in psychoanalytic

[9] Reference footnote 8, Chapter III, especially p. 111. See E. Fromm, *Escape from Freedom*, New York: 1941, for an alternative construction of the psyche in sociocultural process, especially the Appendix, pp. 277–299, for his notion of social character that modifies the physiology and individualism of classical psychoanalysis.

theory and therapy. The quest for universal laws has been surrendered, and we are no longer compelled to force the interpretation of ancient myths to suit empirically disparate facts.

In brief, then, Freud's method suffered from the defects of the reductive, monistic* and exclusively historical approach. It was an achievement of Freud's theoretic ingenuity to have satisfied the demands of all three considerations with his theory of infantile sexuality. It is clear that he used his observations of infantile sexual behavior to uphold reductionism: larger complex wholes of experience were seen and analyzed in terms of their constituent elements; to uphold monism: one single element was held accountable for the varieties of human disturbance and also served as a principle of interpretation; and historicism: the vicissitudes of this one element in early childhood provided all of the necessary data to explain the emergence of difficulties in later life-epochs. The historian of science can interpret the incorporation of these leading principles into his conceptual approach by virtue of the fact that they suffused the intellectual climate of opinion created by Hegel, Marx, Darwin and others, or the philosopher of science may demonstrate how Freud's leading principles fell in line with the scientific determinism and cause-and-effect concatenation of events which pervaded the work of these men. But the student of psychoanalytic therapy who confines himself to psychological methods of treatment can also attribute it to the initial success which Freud had experienced with hysterical patients using Breuer's cathartic method. And this last point will be developed in the next chapter.

The serious criticisms to which Freud's metapsychology has been subjected make it desirable to review his therapeutic conceptions very carefully. The most recent reconstructions have centered their focus largely on his metapsychology. Since theory and practice are closely related to each other, a twin reconstruction of his therapeutic conceptions is required in order to complete the circle. For it seems that Freud's critics have tackled the issues in the following way: They unconsciously accepted the unity of theory and practice on principle, developed practical measures

* See, below, *Addendum* (1964), p. 20.

on the basis of a new frame of reference, and then proceeded to
revise the overarching metapsychological theories. The new therapeutic approaches have not been confronted with the old, however.

There are many unclarities and hiatuses in Freud's writings on
the therapeutic study of transference. This is much more evident
in his earlier writings, especially in his five lectures at Clark University in 1910 where his searching and indecision stand out in
very sharp relief.[10] In his later writings we begin to lose sight of
Freud the searching scientist, and find him making more concerted efforts at final statements. But his final formulations about
the theory of transference fell far short of the actual facts under
clinical observation.[11] The central oversight was that he had per-
mitted the claims of his early work with hysterical patients to
endure in his later therapeutic conceptions. It was a most fortu-
nate circumstance for the history of psychological therapy that
Anna O. was a patient who could easily be hypnotized. But the
concomitant effects of this good fortune did not bode well for the
development of psychoanalysis because when Freud finally discarded hypnotism as a procedure, he persistently recreated its
essential features in the analytic situation.

Today we understand human relationships in a wider sense
than Freud did, and this wider understanding has enabled us
to work through transference situations with greater self-awareness and success. The major shift in our thinking and working
with transference manifestations has come about through the accumulation of analytic experience and the infiltration of knowledge from bordering disciplines, chiefly from cultural anthropology, social psychology and philosophy of science. More concretely,
this shift may be spelled out as follows: Freud treated transference phenomena as specific instances of the repetition-compulsion
which could be traced back to oedipal and pre-oedipal traumata

10 S. Freud, "The Origin and Development of Psychoanalysis," in J. S. Van
Teslaar (ed.), *An Outline of Psychoanalysis*, New York: 1925, pp. 21–70.

11 S. Freud, *A General Introduction to Psychoanalysis*, Garden City: 1943,
Chapter XXVII.

in order to recapture the forgotten episodes and learn more about them. This knowledge, it soon became clear, made little emotional difference in the patient's functioning personality structure. Such intellectual understanding had limited therapeutic value, and the most important thing it probably could do was to reassure the analyst that his metapsychological theory of human development embraced another individual who did not refute it.

Recent trends in psychoanalysis construe the nature and function of transference differently. The current aim is to demonstrate that transference distortions, whatever they happen to be, are reactions to factors which could not have been experienced entirely in the analytic situation. The focus is largely on immediate distortions involving the analyst because "here and now" experiences are currently considered the context of personality change.

Our domain of inquiry is the total personality in action, with current activities and future expectations as much a part of that domain as past experience, remembered or not. Transference distortions are seen essentially as reactions to factors not open to immediate observation. Since the role of these factors cannot be determined apriori, the examination of actual functions and expected consequences has to supplement the exclusive preoccupation with early experience, its communicated content and symbolic value. If we follow this lead, resistance need no longer be conceived as serving nothing but the repression of intolerable memories. In addition to this reference to the past, it also acquires a future reference in perception and imagination. It has, as such, both the positive function of keeping distracting goals out of immediate awareness and the negative function of keeping desirable ends-in-view repressed. That transference and resistance also obscure the vision necessary for the construction of life-goals, the courage necessary for their projection and the appropriate activities for their realization can no longer be ignored.

In short, transference is now considered the major therapeutic instrument which makes psychoanalysis a meaningful emotional undertaking, and therefore transference, resistance and repression are now conceived and applied in a much wider framework.

Roughly speaking, there are five stages in the growth of psychoanalytic technique in studying transference. Freud's first procedure was taken over from Breuer; it aimed to bring about reproduction and abreaction of the "strangulated affect" of the disturbance with the aid of hypnosis. And his two basic changes were essentially changes in procedure. After hypnosis was discarded, his chief technique was to concentrate on the patient's associations and to infer what had not been recalled. In this method of treatment resistances were overcome first by the pressure procedure in which he placed his hands on the patient's forehead and later by interpretation. Finally Freud abandoned concentration on any particular factor or problem and pursued whatever occupied the patient at any particular time with evenly distributed attention. While he continued to interpret resistances in this last procedure, the recollection and interconnection of forgotten episodes were now left to the patient. In this third stage of the evolution Freud took repetition into account for the first time, but its significance as a subject matter for analysis remained to be understood. And the participation of the analyst as a person in his own right was never clearly understood because transference distortions were interpreted mainly in terms of the patient's early oedipal experiences.

The next developments in psychoanalytic technique were not given to Freud to evolve. The analysis of repetitive patterns of feeling, attitude and behavior as evidenced in transference distortions did not come into being until Reich's work on character analysis and A. Freud's work on ego-defenses. And the latest development in technique is the operational or genetic-functional approach—the inclusion of future goals and expectations, that is the category of purpose, in the study of transference distortions.

The decision to abandon recollection as the sole descriptive aim of analysis marks the chief break in this development. Freud's outlook was limited by an unswerving adherence to the aims of hypnosis, and the upshot of it was that he could not take psycho-analysis any further than he did. That his method of psycho-analysis grew out of his early work in hypnotic psychotherapy is widely recognized today. The fact that it was designed to achieve the aims of hypnosis with even greater success has not as yet received the equal recognition it deserves.

It is instructive to note how Fenichel, the acknowledged codifier of Freudian views, defines the transference phenomenon: "The patient misunderstands the present in terms of the past; and, then, instead of remembering the past, he strives, without recognizing the nature of his action, to relive the past and to live it more satisfactorily than he did in childhood." [12] In response to this concise definition our questions about Freud's concept may easily be summarized. Is it merely a misunderstanding that constitutes the transference? Does reliving the past automatically mean that it is an exclusively childhood distortion which is being relived? Will a corrective understanding of the remembered past suffice to clarify its functions in and differences from the present? Is it not also necessary to encompass something of the nature of the present to illuminate the utilization of the past unwittingly? And finally, what is the psychotherapeutic utility of considering transference, resistance and repression without some reference to the category of purpose, aim or goal—that is, without explicit reference to future expectation? These questions have been developed in part through analytic work the objective of which is personality reconstruction, in part because of the results of investigations in scientific fields adjacent to the field of interpersonal processes, and in part by a conception of human experience that is neither monistic, reductive nor value-free.

To answer these questions an extensive review of Freud's technical formulations was undertaken. It soon became astonishingly clear that no aspect of his conception of transference was free of hypnotic traces in theory or practice. And since contemporary technical formulations had not taken this matter into account,

12 O. Fenichel, *The Psychoanalytic Theory of Neurosis*, New York: 1945, p. 29.

the conception of transference had to be revised explicitly developing it.

In reviewing the relevant materials on the subject, we were continually confronted with the fact that its roots were to be found in late nineteenth-century hypnotherapy. And many of the central features of its early formulation—as already noted in Fenichel's definition—grew out of these very same roots. This coincidence has made it possible to present the different facets of our topic without infringing upon the requirements of coherence and unity which a study of this sort deserves.

[*Addendum* (1964): The monism being attributed to Freud's system is explicitly the use of libido theory as his main guide to the formulation of psychoanalytic procedure in his 1915-1917 *Introductory Lectures*, especially in Chapter XXVII and in Chapter XXVIII. His metapsychology, of course, was dualistic throughout, being a dialectic of self-preservative and ego instincts first, and one of eros and thanatos later. Thus, attribution of monism to his therapeutic conceptions requires a firm distinction between metapsychology and psychology (see B. Wolstein, *Freedom to Experience*, New York: 1964, Chapter I). Otherwise, those who interpret Freudianism to mean dualism of eros and thanatos in both metapsychology and psychology are left with a double edged problem: either to explain why Freud omitted thanatos from his conceptions of therapeutic procedure, or attempt a reinterpretation of psychoanalytic procedure to reflect its new-found significance; in any case, the fact remains that Freud's conception of procedure was monistic, reflecting the sexual theory and development of personality in significant phases of the therapeutic effort. Also, see *Appendix A* (1964), p. 214, fn. 7.]

chapter two

Hypnotic Roots

IT MAY BE TRUE that the convergence of psychoanalysis with America's radically different cultural and scientific traditions had crucial significance for the further development of technique and systematics. But it is also true that this sort of sociology of knowledge omits the consideration of internal factors in the development of scientific methodology, and consequently deprives psychoanalysis of its status as an organized method of inquiry and disciplined technique of therapy. Freud's great reliance on the analyst's authority in the treatment situation may be attributed to factors other than his early training in hypnosis; for example, that he was personally an authoritarian, a victim of puritanic ethics or a leading figure in the science and philosophy of modern German thought. To concern ourselves chiefly with such factors seems, however, to gloss over the persistent influence of hypnosis on the evolution and practice of classic analytic technique. Freud was a profound student of human psychology, bent on creating a sound therapeutic technique, and his early acceptance of hypnotic method as well as his eventual failure to free himself from its confining aims cannot be understood without placing them in this latter context.

The history of hypnosis from Mesmer to Breuer and Freud has already been recorded and documented.[1] These two men made outstanding innovations in hypnotic psychotherapy which, if taken alone, would have earned an important place in the history of psychological treatment for both of them: Breuer's cathartic method which worked well with hysterics, and Freud's technique of free association, his systematic interpretation of dreams, his discoveries of repression, resistance, transference.

These latter discoveries which Freud rightly considered the

[1] L. R. Wolberg, *Medical Hypnosis*, Volume I, New York: 1948, Chapter I.

foundations of psychoanalytic therapy had not, however, been disentangled from their original matrix. What Freud had done was to dispense with some of the accidental features of hypnosis whose effectiveness proved unsatisfactory. He gradually developed his method of psychoanalysis to remedy this situation, but it was essentially a difference in the procedure rather than in the goal of treatment. Transference, for him, was but another name for suggestibility; resistance replaced the type and depth of hypnotic trance necessary for making the patient's suggestibility accessible; and the analytic concern with repression of early events duplicated the primary goal of recollection in hypnosis. He thought that his chief contribution to the understanding of transference was his libido theory, his sexual explanation of suggestibility. But when he presented it in its final form, he had to devote the large part of a lecture to this point in response to questions which were raised at the end of the previous one.[2] How much clearer this sexual theory of personality development made the coordinate processes of suggestion and suggestibility is still a debatable point; we will have to return to it.

The original cathartic method was developed by Breuer in order to abrogate "the efficacy of the original non-abreacted ideas, affording an outlet to their strangulated affects through speech."[3] The goal, then, was the reconstruction and abreaction of the repressed past. Breuer believed that almost all psychological symptoms originated as remnants of affectively tinged experiences in the ancient past; for that reason they were later called psychic traumata. In catharsis, he found that symptoms of hysterical disturbance would disappear when the hypnotized patient could be made to remember the traumatic situation in which they first appeared. Such recall was effective if the resurrected emotions were given free rein. The historically significant thing about cathartic therapy is that no one had ever attempted to cure hysteri-

2 S. Freud, *A General Introduction to Psychoanalysis*, Garden City: 1943, Chapters XXVII and XXVIII.

3 J. Breuer and S. Freud, *Studies in Hysteria*, New York: 1936, p. 12. This theoretic statement of the matter was a product of their joint efforts.

cal symptoms by such means before, and no one had made this attempt with a strictly psychological explanation of their etiology. Breuer's cathartic method elicited and sustained the unconscious dependencies of Anna O. Yet his method differed from that of classical analysis as it was finally developed. He did not confuse the patient's current feelings with an all too ready interpretation of them in terms of a repetition-compulsion which started in infancy.[4] The discovery of the effectiveness of catharsis was, in a sense, the profound contribution of Anna O. Breuer had modified the established authoritarian technique with a more permissive one: he was willing to listen to her views and feelings about her disturbing experiences. Of course, we will never know whether it was necessary to rely on unconscious dependencies and the hypnotic trance in her case. But we do know that neither is necessarily required of the patient for effective psychoanalytic therapy to take place and that the former can be analyzed when they persist in the guise of a positive transference.

Thus, despite Breuer's permissiveness, his procedure did not encompass the analysis of Anna O.'s unconscious dependencies which are now considered a distortion. The fact that she may not have been ready to enter into an equalitarian relationship at the time is beside the point; the essential point is that, in this hypnocathartic procedure of touching off and utilizing unconscious processes for so-called positive therapeutic ends, the unconscious processes have been unwittingly reinforced by the give-and-take with the therapist. And this only makes it more difficult to explore them at some future time. In fact, future interactions with people in general and therapists in particular will take place on

4 S. Rado, "Recent Advances in Psychoanalytic Therapy," in *Proceedings of the Association for Research in Nervous and Mental Disease,* Baltimore: 1953. Seeking to distinguish Freud from Breuer, Rado has stressed that Breuer appears to have been a more permissive person and to have allowed his patient the psychological room she required to talk openly about her repressed rage. Yet, his criticisms of Freud's therapeutic procedure with positive transference apply with equal force to Breuer's hypnocathartic procedure. Compare I. Macalpine, "The Development of the Transference," *Psychoanalytic Quarterly,* XIX (1950), pp. 501–539.

the tacit assumption that the unresolved dependency distortions will be accepted and accommodated at face value rather than explored and understood as patterns of distortion.

This reliance on unresolved dependency in hypnotic therapy of any sort—prohibitive, supportive or cathartic—limits the utility of this method of treatment so far as contemporary psychoanalysis is concerned. Some analysts may want to retain it in their treatment repertoire for whatever emergency situations they encounter, but all hypnotic attempts are ruled out of a psychoanalytic method which has self-reliant behavior as its therapeutic goal. Breuer's technique did not achieve it because he required the persistence of Anna O.'s dependency problems in order that the cathartic experience set in.

Freud soon came to dislike this method of therapy. In the first place he did not like the magical connotations surrounding hypnosis. Secondly, and perhaps more important, it also became evident that he could not hypnotize all of his patients by any means; so he changed Breuer's method and made the cathartic phase independent of hypnotism. This innovation, on the face of it, confronted him with the apparently senseless and impossible task of trying to learn something from the patient which neither the patient nor the analyst knew. He proceeded none the less to work with his patients in their normal state because of what he had once been taught by Bernheim, the great French investigator of hypnosis. Bernheim had demonstrated that hypnotic subjects did not really forget their hypnotic experiences. He could awaken memories of these experiences after the subjects had returned to their normal state. Even if they said at first that they did not remember, he persisted, urged and assured them they did know what was in the shadows of amnesia, and they were able to recall the hypnotic suggestion or command.

How Freud adapted this experiment of Bernheim's is clear from his own case of Emmy von N.: "As is customary in hypnotic psycho-therapy, I combatted the existing morbid ideas through assurances, prohibitions, and the introduction of all kinds of counter ideas, but I was not satisfied with just that. I traced, therefore, the history of the origin of the individual symptoms in order to be able to combat the assumptions upon which the morbid ideas were constructed . . . How much of each therapeutic result could be attributed to this suggesting away in *statu nascendi,* and how much to the loosening of the affect through abreaction I cannot state." [5] Though written back in 1889, this is an important statement because it illustrates Freud's early concern with resistance to repressed memories and his attempt to resolve conflicts by using suggestion, prohibition and all kinds of counter ideas.

When Freud first separated the cathartic phase of hypnocathartic therapy from hypnosis, he introduced the pressure procedure to facilitate the production of memories he considered necessary for the understanding of the symptom. This pressure procedure was first described in the Case of Lucy R.[6] and it was first applied in the Case of Elizabeth v. R.[7] When the patient had reached the point in her associations where she knew nothing more, Freud would assure her that she did know and must reveal it; in fact at the moment he placed his hand on her forehead the right memory would emerge. In this way he succeeded, without the direct aid of hypnosis, to prove that forgotten memories were not lost, just as Bernheim had shown at Nancy that hypnotic experiences could be recalled in the normal state under pressure. He soon observed, however, that the pressure procedure was hardly adequate. It worked the first time it was used, and ideas subsequently emerged which had little or no connection with the purpose at hand; not only the therapist but even the patient herself would reject them as incorrect.

In response to this state of affairs, he turned to the method of free association on the assumption that incorrect and useless ideas for the context under investigation only seemed to be useless and incorrect. Although they seemed to emerge inappropriately, they were taken as surrogates of the repressed traumata—new, artifi-

5 Reference footnote 3, p. 73.
6 Reference footnote 3, p. 79.
7 Reference footnote 3, pp. 109–110.

cial, ephemeral, disguised, yet somehow connected with the memories under search; and it was postulated that the degree of disguise was the barometer of resistance to the emergence of this or that idea. If only the patient abided by the fundamental rule of free association and communicated her thoughts as they occurred, there would be a good prospect for uncovering the underlying constellation of traumatic situations and feelings. This was so on the belief that nothing can occur and be reported without having some sort of bearing on the repressed complex of experiences the analyst is seeking—a belief which has been seriously shaken by recent analytic work with the intellectual meanderings of obsessive people who can talk to the point of boredom without saying much of anything meaningful about their difficulties.

An analytic therapy subscribing to the view that everything the patient says or does has some bearing on his difficulty, however remote, must also maintain that associating ideas is anything but free. Free association, it may be pointed out in passing, was a misnomer at best, for the associative processes were believed to be anything but random. In Freud's view, the interconnection of the expressed surrogate and the repressed complex was actually overdetermined.

By the time Freud published his Case of Dora psychoanalytic technique had been completely revolutionized. The method in the *Studies in Hysteria,* of starting with the symptoms and clearing them up one after another, had already been discarded. The analysis of symptoms one by one had the tantalizing qualities of a chameleon. To arrange a final and decisive encounter with the core of any one symptom was found to be impossible. When any single one was approached, it became transformed into another, and the therapeutic process was turned into a continual see-saw to which there could be no satisfactory termination. "Since then," he wrote in 1905, "I have abandoned that technique, because I find it totally inadequate for dealing with the finer structure of a neurosis. I now let the patient himself choose the subject of the day's work, and in that way I start out from whatever surface his unconscious happens to be presenting to his notice at the moment. But on this plan everything that has to do with the clearing-up of a particular symptom emerges piecemeal, woven into various contexts, and distributed over widely separated periods of time. In spite of this apparent disadvantage . . . there can be no doubt that it (the new technique) is the only possible one." [8]

This view of the matter is certainly a valid one today. Though enunciated nearly fifty years ago, it cannot be changed because it highlights the importance of seeing the various symptoms in the context of the total personality. No particular symptom can be intensively examined as a separate entity because it is interwoven in the various contexts which have to be followed in their multiple dimensions; and no symptom can be analyzed and resolved apart from the total personality organization. And it also declares the implicit surrender of suggestive therapy: for if a symptom were successfully suggested away in one context, it would reappear in other contexts, disguised and on the face of it a new symptom calling for singular treatment by the old method.

For the student of Freud's writings, however, this early statement creates more problems than it solves because it leaves us without a consistent position to attribute to him. We shall soon see that he considered the transference phenomenon a return to the power of suggestion and that he had no clear-cut distinction between hypnotic suggestion and suggestion in transference. But it may be pointed out here that he had not even surrendered symptom analysis finally and irrevocably. For when we turn to his final discussion of therapeutic technique in 1918, we find that the libido of the neurotic was attached to the symptoms which provided substitutive gratifications; and the therapeutic objective was to dissolve the symptoms by going back to their point of origin, reviewing the conflict from which they developed and guiding the conflict to a new resolution with the help of psychological forces which were not available at that time.[9] Here we

8 S. Freud, "Fragment of an Analysis of a Case of Hysteria," *Collected Papers*, Volume III, London: 1925, p. 19.

9 Reference footnote 2, p. 395.

see that symptom analysis was still practiced, though the technique of symptom analysis had been expressly discarded some
thirteen years earlier. The striking thing about this reversal in
judgment is that Freud made it in the name of the new and revolutionized procedure of psychoanalysis, his final technical point
of view. In fact this last quotation, if its source were not noted,
could just as easily have been read as early as 1889 in his case
study of Emmy von N.

Freud developed his theory of transference about ten years after
he had separated cathartic method from hypnosis. He had arrived at it without the use of hypnotic technique. He evidently
recognized that hypnosis obscured and obviated the operation of
resistances in order to get at the repressions straightaway, that it
made a certain part of the mental field freely accessible only by
concealing the system of resistances from the interpersonal relationship of therapist and patient. And he even realized that resistances on the borders of this accessible field accumulated in a
way that made what was beyond them inaccessible during the
hypnotic trance. It may, at first blush, seem curious that he continued to seek recall of the past—the goal of hypnotism—even
after he had discerned these grave defects. But this makes sense
when seen against the fact that Freud's psychoanalytic method
was geared not so much to elucidate the fabric of interpersonal
processes but rather to excavate the traumata of early childhood.
The idea that nothing is forgotten, which he had derived from
his work with Bernheim and Breuer, was translated into the dictum that everything had to be remembered for constructive analytic therapy.

Thus far I have tried to demonstrate a continuous line of development through the three stages in Freud's development of
psychoanalytic technique. It leads back as a single thread to the
early orientation in hypnotic technique—that is, the quest for
forgotten episodes of the past and dealing with the patient's defenses against recalling them. There were many points of similarity throughout. The belief in the strict determination of mental
events was shared by hypnosis and psychoanalysis; it conferred

a sense of absolute certainty on the therapeutic quest for self-knowledge, and produced an air of dogmatic authority in the therapeutic relationship. Freud carried over this firm reliance on the therapist's authority, which may definitely be traced to hypnotic psychotherapy, into his final development of analytic technique. The paramount need to struggle with resistance, already postulated in Bernheim's and Breuer's methods, was continued by Freud even after he had introduced the pressure procedure because some patients were not hypnotizable. Yet after dropping both hypnosis and the pressure procedure, he "gained the impression that through urging alone it would really be impossible to bring to light the definitely existing pathogenic series of ideas. . . . I, therefore, formulated this whole state of affairs into the following theory: *Through my psychic work I had to overcome a psychic force in the patient which opposed the pathogenic ideas from becoming conscious (remembered).*" [10] And this is essentially the point he was to make in 1918 in his first introductory lectures to the effect that the analyst calls upon all of his available resources in order to bring the patient to another decision. He saw the transference relationship as a battlefield on which the contending forces had to clash.[11] The dominant concern was with the forgotten past; and the postulated need to struggle with the patient was pursued with full knowledge that either the therapist emerged victorious, which was called a positive affectionate transference or the patient resisted treatment which was a negative hostile transference—these characteristics of hypnosis were translated into fundamental principles of classical psychoanalysis. Freud accepted them quite early in his career and never surrendered their perspective on the interaction of therapist and patient.

That Freud's contribution was first and foremost a procedural one and that his changes did not affect the aim of hypnotic therapy or its idea of recovery cannot be stressed too strongly. He never vacillated about it despite the many changes in his new

[10] Reference footnote 3, p. 201.
[11] Reference footnote 2, p. 395.

psychotherapeutic approach. This new approach was in fact a better avenue to that original hypnotic aim, and he never ventured beyond this definition of his field of inquiry. In one place, his statement was very explicit: *"The aim of these different procedures has of course remained the same throughout:* descriptively, to recover lost memories; dynamically, to conquer the resistances caused by repression." [12] These were the descriptive and dynamic goals of hypnosis as well as of psychoanalysis as Freud perfected it, while the difference, as he saw it, was merely procedural.

And it must be noted that when he took repetitions in behavior into account, it was to further these descriptive and dynamic aims: "There are cases which under the new technique conduct themselves up to a point like those under the hypnotic technique and only later abandon this behavior; but others behave differently from the beginning . . . we may say that here the patient *remembers* nothing of what is forgotten and repressed, but that he expresses it in *action* . . . he *repeats* it, without of course knowing that he is repeating it." [13] Because he had not freed himself from the hypnotic vestiges of recollection and resistance to recollection, the compulsion to repeat became but another source of factual material which was enacted without being remembered. In fact, even transference was also seen as "only a bit of repetition . . . the transference of the forgotten past." [14] The compulsion to repeat was first and foremost a substitute for the impulse to remember, and the therapeutic task cut out for analysis was to reduce the one into the other—an important phase of the work but certainly not the entire job.

But Freud easily justified his procedure by appeal to the unrelinquished aim of hypnosis. "Recollection in the old style," he wrote, "reproduction in the mind, remains the goal of his (the analyst's) endeavors. . . . When the transference has developed

[12] S. Freud, "Further Recommendations in the Technique of Psychoanalysis," *Collected Papers*, Volume II, London: 1924, p. 367, italics added.

[13] Reference footnote 9, p. 369.

[14] Reference footnote 9, p. 370.

to a sufficiently strong attachment, the treatment is in a position to prevent all the more important of the patient's repetition-actions and to make use of his intentions alone, *in statu nascendi,* as material for the therapeutic work." [15] Though Freud recognized "that it is only by dire experience that mankind ever learns sense," [16] he also seems to have retained the idea that the problem was to be treated *in statu nascendi,* for reproduction in the mind was still the desirable state. But more important for the purposes of our theme, he still considered it necessary to reproduce the conditions of hypnosis even after he had expressly given up its method. Here again, just as the authority of the hypnotist was primary during the induction and course of the trance, so the psychoanalyst exercised authority to control the course of the analysis; the patient had to reproduce his problem in the mind and promise to forswear important decisions during the course of treatment—the decision on importance being left presumably to the analyst—though he was not hindered from realizing "foolish projects" [17] of no special significance.

This idea of reproduction in the mind has to be qualified for therapeutic application. If put into effect at the very beginning of an analysis, it places on the analyst the unwelcome burden of deciding that certain aspects of the patient's personality are distortions and that they have to be inhibited in advance of knowledge. It also places on the patient an equally unfair burden of having to inhibit behavior of which he knows neither the motives nor the rationale for inhibiting it. The analyst is no infallible deity who can divine the psychological source of any particular patient's difficulty; nor is the patient a robot who can consistently maintain a mechanical mode of performance without insight and understanding. Where the evidence is clear-cut that the behavior is producing irretrievable damage in the patient's life, there is little question about it; and, under such circumstances, the ambulatory patient's cooperation is usually obtained

[15] Reference footnote 12, p. 373.
[16] Reference footnote 12, p. 373.
[17] Reference footnote 12, p. 373.

with ease. But quite a period of analytic inquiry is ordinarily needed before the analyst can discern harmful effects of distortions, before the patient has done sufficient work to get some glimmerings of the significant unconscious processes.

To insist on the reproduction of conflictual factors exclusively in the mind duplicates one of the characteristics of hypnosis in psychoanalysis. This may not be a serious objection in itself, but to insist on it in advance of knowledge will actually deprive the patient of other bases for learning about the unconscious processes involved in his difficulties; and it can lead to the further contraction of his sense of self-esteem. This insistence may have been motivated by Freud's desire to avoid the ill-effects of acting out conflicts in therapy and life. But it is fraught with the danger of limiting both experience and resolution of problems to the analyst's denotation of them. Of course, the analyst with sufficient training and skill may often be right in his calculation of the problem, but if the patient does not have an opportunity to make his own observations and conclusions, then he must take the analyst's judgment on blind faith or authoritative suggestion of the "analyst knows best" variety. For this sort of thing to work, there is usually a positive transference in existence which carries decidedly distorted elements within itself. And when it does work under such conditions, it leaves unresolved the problem of the patient's all too ready suggestibility.

This conception has of course changed. Current or expected actions are also considered an important source of knowledge about transference, resistance and repression; and the anxiety accompanying them is now at the center of therapeutic interest. The vestiges of hypnotic psychotherapy which had captured Freud's imagination and perspective quite early in his work probably prevented him from using current actions and future expectations and the resistances to them as equally important points of reference for studying the repetitions in behavior.

In order to understand Freud's development of psychoanalytic technique, it is necessary to see that he never surrendered the hypnotic conception of treatment. In his second series of introductory lectures, he asserted that he had "discussed the theoretical side of the subject (therapeutic aspect of psychoanalysis) fifteen years ago, and I cannot formulate it in any other way today." [18] And "fifteen years ago" would date his first series of *Introductory Lectures* in 1915–1917. This rather interesting assertion points up the fact that his therapeutic conceptions were not affected by the many theoretic innovations of the intervening years. There were many basic reformulations during those years. Most important of all from a therapeutic standpoint was the drastic revision of his views on neurotic symptoms in 1926: strangulated affects of early traumatic experiences were no longer the chief cause of neurosis, and even though neurotic symptoms still served the dual purpose of crystallizing repressed instinctual forces and representing defenses against them, he reversed his position on the nature of anxiety; he now held that anxiety never arose from repressed libido.[19] At about this time there was also a drastic revision of his instinct theory in which the death instinct was set forth for the first time. Yet, despite these and other major systematic changes, Freud saw no need to revise any of his therapeutic conceptions in his *New Lectures* of 1933, or in later publications.[20]

[18] S. Freud, *New Introductory Lectures on Psychoanalysis*, London: 1933, pp. 206–207.

[19] S. Freud, *The Problem of Anxiety*, New York: 1936, p. 51. Though it is not always easy to be certain about Freud's views in this outstanding study, it is an exciting intellectual event when a man in his sixties does not hesitate to reverse himself on views which were beyond any shadow of doubt only a few years before.

[20] In his outstanding paper of 1937, "Analysis Terminable and Interminable," *Collected Papers*, Volume V, London: 1950, pp. 316–357,. Freud continued to modify his libido theory, holding now that changes in ego structure have an etiology independent of the strength of the instincts (pp. 321–322) ; that instinctual conflict can be described more accurately as a conflict between the ego and an instinct (p. 324) ; and that resolutions of personality conflict in later stages of personality development are to be taken into account as "after-repressions" (p. 328) . But he developed this idea of "after-repression"

Without a definite realization that the hypnotic roots of his therapeutic conceptions were not affected by these later theoretic revisions the meaning and context of his last views about transference and resistance would remain vague. And the import of later developments in the technique of analytic therapy would, moreover, become unintelligible.

---

side by side with the notion that there are no fresh repressions in later years because the old ones persist and appear over and over again in different conflict situations.

Thus the recall of the early past was still retained as a goal of psychoanalysis in the same way that it was a goal in hypnosis. I have not been able to find a frank and direct renunciation of the position taken in 1914—see reference footnote 12 above—in any of Freud's writings.

chapter three

Early Trauma or Total Personality

FREUD'S VERY EARLY VIEWS about rapport and transference were predicated on an oversimplified notion: certain specific forgotten memories, traumatically embedded in the unconscious, had to be recaptured, and this would purge the mind of the disturbing factors that produced symptoms. The original source of this notion was clearly hypnosis, the best therapeutic method to accomplish such a task. His later formulations about the structure of mind were developed after he had completed his work on transference analysis. The new mental topography did not, strangely enough, prompt him to alter his therapeutic conceptions. Since Anna Freud's and Reich's contributions to the understanding of ego and character defenses, we know that a complicated personality structure has intervened between the postulated forgotten memories of early childhood and the contemporary disturbances. And this field of inquiry has replaced the dominant concern with isolated and possibly single incidents in the forgotten past.

The total personality in action is now the focus in which we study the meaning of psychological disturbance. Its habitual modes of adaptation are conceived and demonstrated as effects and developments in an interpersonal field which is organized to cope with typical expectancies, real or distorted. Hence hypnosis is not an appropriate technique or therapy, since it bypasses these subsequent effects and contemporary developments. Its express purpose is to circumvent the intervening personality organization and to establish comparatively direct inroads on the past. It has limited applicability as a method of research and therapy just because of this direct access to the past, and so the exclusive pursuit of its goals can only exert a restrictive influence on the analytic process. At the present stage of our knowledge, the only psychotherapeutic technique which encompasses distortions in the entire range of personality development is the operational or genetic-functional analysis of transference.

Let us suppose that the single early trauma can be recovered through the patient's herculean feats of memory or at the instance of the analyst's concerted pressures—then what? The patient is still left with the selfsame recurrences in his everyday life which cannot be understood and broken through simply in terms of a single event at a single point in the remote excavated past. This type of procedure has an abstract intellectual motif running through it because the patient will never again have that singular interpersonal integration with the person or persons involved at that time. And unless the analyst is particularly pressuring and forces the data to fit his theoretic framework, he will be hard pressed to convince the patient that it is that specific event which repeated itself in all of the many different interpersonal encounters since that original traumatic event. If that single early trauma can be recaptured, well and good; it takes its place as one in the series of instances we study in their relevant specifics. If that early episode cannot be recaptured, it is equally good, for current patterns of integration provide sufficient information to occupy us for quite a long time in analysis. There is no substitute for the close and continuous study of recurring reactions, present as well as past, if we want to obtain a meaningful understanding of their probable future course.

The inclusion of current actions, future expectations and resistance to their consequences seems to follow logically from the liberation of psychoanalysis from the relentless quest for lost memories. This latter goal was Freud's exclusive concern because his view of personality development was mechanical and deterministic; and the converse would be equally true, that he constructed such a theory of personality development in order to establish the fixed and schematic elements of those early experiences in later life. The study of current problems, from this perspective, became a mere formality. The patient's consecutive movements through a series of situations simply provided duplications of the infantile experiences, and such duplications could be reduced to their early prototypical state and be considered as merely having been repeated without basic change. There was posited an original event or set of events which repeated itself throughout one's life-course basically unchanged—whatever that would mean—and if only we were to ferret out its forgotten basis, it would not have to be repeated at all. If this assumption were not made, Freud's entire enterprise would make little sense in its own terms; and it implies that he made his technical advances in spite of his early and continued allegiance to the aims of hypnotic therapy.

Once these mechanistic implications for personality development are reconstructed, however, this one-sided approach need not encumber the final therapeutic procedure which he evolved. Instead of satisfying the apriori conditions imposed by hypnotic treatment, the method may follow the lead of the subject matter and determine its own conditions of operation.

The repetition-compulsion, in Freud's conceptual system, denies the fact of emergence, novelty and reconstructability, since its mechanistic formulation located the possibilities for change in the initial events of a developmental series. It was construed as being solely a property of a traumatic event or set of events located at single points in time in a particular era of personality development—the oedipal phase or earlier. This deterministic view makes the very possibility of psychoanalytic therapy theoretically dubious; it seems, moreover, to reverse the actualities of the case, since the compulsion to repeat, as we know today, evolves very gradually and continually undergoes some modicum of change, if only the slightest, in each of the multiple situations in which it occurs. The compulsion to repeat need no longer be analyzed as a mechanical repetition. It may be conceived as a habitual interpersonal pattern whose future is open-ended, as a dynamic mode of reaction which has evolved, perhaps lost its original reason for being, and emerged with new and different functions requiring independent examination. For the emergence of a repetition, being woven into a variety of dissimilar situations over widely distributed periods of time, acquires new features which must also be treated in their own terms.

And it need not be assumed that the infantile problem has always remained one and the same throughout. Such an assumption eliminates the very fact of change from the process which the patient presumably wants to change. In fact, if we did make it, we would put the analyst in that peculiar position of offering to provide services which he had implicitly declared himself unable to provide in the first place. The psychological fact seems to be that people change all of the time whether they are in analytic therapy or not; and these perhaps hardly noticeable modifications which are always occurring provide the analyst with opening wedges to define the problem in a useful way.

Interpersonal processes are not only stable, they are also plastic; they are not only recurrent, they are also emergent; they not only reproduce the old, they also reconstruct it in new and changing ways. When I use the concept of repetition in this essay, its meaning is intended to convey both kinds of qualities— at once stable and plastic, recurrent and emergent, reproductive and reconstructive. And of special importance: when a repetition is about to be carried out, it is not only automatic but it also holds the potentiality of being suspended in mid-action. In not having already been done, it may not need to be done or undone. In the realm of the future it is still a hypothetical act, probable and anticipated on the basis of past experience; but not being fully necessary nor predetermined, it may yet incorporate new characteristics just as it has always incorporated them in the face of what were once unlived experiences. The meaning of the concept of repetition is thus enlarged by the inclusion of current actions and future experience.

Now scientists use probability in order to represent and predict the frequent repetition of an occurrence; this is true for physics as well as statistical psychology and sociology. In psychoanalysis, transference phenomena alone provide us with the significant data on probability of reaction, the assumption being that modes of response over which the patient has no control are repeated in the interpersonal experience with the analyst and that they usually have a high frequency in the patient's general interpersonal relations. This can be checked by asking the patient whether he has had such an experience before, with whom, under what circumstances and to what ends. Furthermore, if the transference distortion is a major one, these inquiries on the part of the analyst may be rewarded with a series of situations in the past and present and even in the expected future which exhibit the same regularity. The distortion is thus considered to be a repeated form of behavior, a habit of misperception which is observed with an especial frequency and which may be attributed to events in the history of that individual. These frequent communications of a misperception are the observable facts which may be studied as such and as embodiments of a certain induplicable event at a certain dubious point in the unknown past. What they are embodiments of remains an open question depending on the metapsychological orientation of the particular analyst; and this question does not always need to be answered definitively so long as frequent patterns of reaction are mastered and greater freedom and understanding are enjoyed.

Many of the technical terms of psychoanalysis point to a powerful theoretic and therapeutic interest in repetition-reactions as its subject matter. We say that someone suffers from "claustrophobia" if he repeatedly becomes uncomfortable in confined places. He is "anal-erotic" if he often finds it necessary to be miserly, rigid or stubborn. He has "sexual phobias" if he frequently finds it impossible to engage in sexual activities; or he has "compulsions" if he frequently engages in any specific sort of behavior over which he has no control. These terms are ad hoc definitions which move the focus of inquiry away from repetitive patterns with observable frequencies to fixed momentary states. But this notion of the momentary present is specious and deceptive; it is neither momentary nor present but an inferred condition about past, present and future. The effect of such terms as phobia, anal-erotism and compulsion adds to the deceptiveness of this inferred condition—that is, instead of studying these diverse phenomena as observable frequencies in their contingencies and individual differences, we translate them into a sort of fixed quality or trait possessed by the personality and we then look for the single significant event at some single point in the past and assign a deterministic status to it.

If we were only concerned with forgotten episodes and utilized the repetitive reactions exhibited in transference simply to awaken memories of early childhood, we would miscalculate the importance of the ongoing repetition-reactions which are touched off by current environing conditions; and we would overlook the possibility for putting the study of these reactions on a sound empirical basis. The forgotten episodes, the search for which Freud began in hypnosis and continued in his final conception of analytic technique, were single events. But since they did not repeat themselves as such, they could not become the proper subject matter of an empirical science; and psychoanalytic psychology would never move beyond the realm of the phenomenological. Events that have already occurred and may never again be repeated ordinarily hold limited interest. But the effects of these events which have an orderly and recurrent pattern can be studied by a descriptive and inferential methodology.

Scientists are usually concerned with the future as well as the past of the subject matter chosen for study. Yet, psychoanalysts also want to know what an individual will do; and we strive to construct hypotheses about some of the features his personality will have under certain specifiable circumstances. But what sort of subject matter is the future of personality organization in psychoanalysis? How is it represented in the communication under observation? It can only be represented in the regularities which are observable or at least subject to inference, and we assume that knowledge of these regularities will develop the power of our patients to control eventual outcomes once they acquire sufficient understanding of the conditions of their occurrence.

Personality denotes a configuration of enduring thoughts and behaviors which confer meaning upon a socialized individual and differentiate him from other members of his group. This term points at once to a generalized construct and to a unique human being. It refers to a generalization with respect to the way in which an enduring configuration of events develops and functions, but it also specifies a particular being with respect to the aims and attitudes encompassed by that pattern. For if personality is defined as a pattern of regularities in experience, then individuality means the uniqueness of what is patterned. Psychoanalytic observation is bifocal, however, and the approach to events as expressed in attitudes and feelings is more significant than the actual events the patient describes. The latter are recurrent situations A, B and C of the construct of personality; the former are the interpersonal processes, the A^n, B^n and C^n, which have accrued to those events. The method here is one of observing how event A is described, observing how attitude A^n is expressed, and inferring accompanying attitudes from the relationships in which the total pattern is expressed and described. Thus the specific activity is not only a part of the behavioral configuration ABC; it is also an overt expression of A^n which is itself part of an intricate system of attitudes and motives. What is most frequent as studied under clinical conditions usually yields the initial evidence about these interpersonal attitudes.

The problem of social psychology as a science is to correlate attitudes and feelings with particular patterns of institutionalized behavior. The problem of psychoanalysis as a therapeutic art is to bring about an awareness of specific disturbances in attitude-behavior relationships so that they become reorganized or relinquished in accordance with the needs of the specific person. Ethics, on the other hand, deals with the comparative evaluations which are placed on these whole units of attitude-behavior. During particular inquiries, these disciplines should not be reduced to each other, and all three must be kept distinct because they are differing emphases in a single range of facts about personality.

Institutional forms of social behavior do not constitute the concrete subject matter of psychotherapeutic inquiry; the psychoanalytic situation is preeminently interpersonal. To be sure, re-current interpersonal processes develop in and through a cultural matrix, but the study of the former is not simply interchange-able with the study of the latter which concentrates on disturb-ances in "me-you" relationships. From a structural point of view, the interpersonal meaning of a transference repetition cannot be established by generalized inquiry into social behavior, for even within a similar structure or pattern of social behavior diverse interpersonal processes are seen to be in operation. Intensive in-quiry into its psychodynamic components within the situation in which it unfolds is required. And this unfolding of psychological processes is studied both historically and functionally—both in-tensively within the immediate present of "befores" and "afters" and extensively into the remembered past and anticipated future, fragmentary or whole. For in a severe psychological disturbance, what is repeated with unusual frequency is usually a defensive operation. Any variation in response or flexibility in reaction is sorely conspicuous by its absence; and intensive analysis is re-quired in order to understand the crystallization of emotional factors of which the repetition is an expression.

The approach presented thus far has only highlighted the kind of result which follows from the view that repetition-reactions, frequent and probable, are the subject matter of psychoanalysis. It has already been noted that the repetition of interpersonal processes is a rather lawful, orderly and patterned fact. Once dis-cerned by observation, description and inference, it becomes an easy fact to work with because its simplicity has striking emo-tional effects. The hold it is able to acquire and maintain on the patient's interest is another clue to its significance. Of course, pa-tients do not always know what is worthy of their interest, but in the event that the analyst's formulation is not meaningful to the patient, there is hardly any working base possible; there is only limited motivational drive, if that. On the other hand, a formulation which can be agreed upon in common as the defini-tion of the analytic problem has the status of a hypothesis which is always subject to modification with the appearance of new data. Sensitive movements into the patient's life are required of the analyst at appropriate levels of motivation. This is done to increase mutual understanding of the meaningful interactions that take place between them. And when the analyst follows the lead of the patient's motivation for cooperative endeavor as a guide to the definition of the disturbance, he contributes to the fruitful and constructive possibilities in psychoanalytic collaboration. Besides, if insight is imposed from without, it will be subject to the fate of all authoritarian dicta: cause the interdicted disturbance to pursue its customary ends in secret, obstruct free expression on future occasions and make it impossible to observe the probable aggravation of the disturbance—the resultant secrecy of the disturbance being itself a contributing factor.

The fact that transference repetitions are easily produced by each new patient embarking upon an analysis makes it possible to take his total personality in action as a subject matter. Because they are readily produced in the analytic situation as well as in day-to-day activities, it is also possible for him to experiment with them in a limited way under observable clinical conditions. If the essential features of a transference reaction, after they have been provisionally defined, are not readily duplicated in a new situation, we do not take it as a cue to resort to statistical averages. It is an indication that some relevant factor has yet to be described and incorporated in a now modified hypothesis. In other words the desired uniformity of results in applying our definition of the transference distortion prompts us to turn not to other situations for exemplification but to a more intensive investigation of the situation already presented by the patient. With the progressive intensification of inquiry the analytic work may then continue to a review of previously reported situations with increasing clarity and precision. The other alternative—to introduce statistical and conceptual manipulation of the data in order to interpret probable origins or results—would only create greater distance between the analyst's interpretations and the patient's experience.

There are three kinds of terms which are used in hypotheses to understand the frequent patterns of interpersonal processes: (1) Those which are susceptible of direct observation even though the process to which they refer is not now observable; this may be illustrated by the assumption of underlying anxiety during a transference distortion, anxiety which is not always demonstrable the first time the hypothesis about it is proferred, though subsequent search may reveal its presence. (2) Those which involve the operation of some process which is assumed in advance to be forever beyond direct observation; they project the many past events which we assume to have happened even though they can no longer be directly observed by anyone, and whether the past events interpreted through these terms have been or can be recalled, the hypotheses about them bring together and correlate propositions regarding currently observable patterns. And (3) those metapsychological terms which are assumed to be forever beyond direct observation because they refer to events or substrates of experience whose unobservability is an intrinsic aspect of their formulation; the purpose of notions like libido, birth trauma, the drive for mental health, the interpersonal origins and functions of character disturbances and so on is chiefly to correlate and explain inferences about observed processes. The application of the first type of hypothetical constructs is most useful for intensifying the investigation of palpably unclear situations, while those of types (2) and (3) are ordinarily avoided except on occasions when a more systematic integration of data is indicated.

It is important to underscore the fact that any intensive study of frequent distortions provides an immediate reference to personal experience. This immediate reference is generally lacking in concepts or laws or any products of logical, experimental or statistical operations. And this cannot be shunted aside as another imperative which psychoanalytic science is trying to impose on its patients. Nor can it be dismissed simply because certain types of patients like nothing better than to fiddle with alternative intellectual explanations of behavior which they have as yet only the remotest intention of changing. The direct study of the repetition in its occurrence confers emotional immediacy on our study of interpersonal processes. Besides, when we seek to extend the results of an analysis to general human behavior, it is a great advantage for psychoanalysis to have a conceptual system which refers to a single individual, preferably without extensive comparisons to the social group. This makes it possible for both patient and analyst to gather and to apply psychoanalytic knowledge more directly.

The study of regularities in transference distortions provides psychoanalysis with an opportunity to obtain a continuous and live account of experience. We can follow the repetition of any distortion into the past and look into its eventual outcomes in the future. This is in marked contrast to Freud's three different procedures which had as their single aim to recover lost memories. If we were to sample the transference distortions from time to time for the sole purpose of ferreting out forgotten memories, we would have to rely on the pressure of inference, in which case the continuity and forward movement of the process would also have to be inferred. And Freud's inferential procedure has also slighted an important facet of human experience—current impulse, desire or drive, within or beyond awareness. Psychoanalytic science may have tried to predict the outcome of a given course of human behavior, but knowledge that predictive value was being accorded to reactions became a crucial factor in the already indeterminate situation. Moreover, awareness of impulse, desire or purpose can change; and such changes made prediction even more fallible.

The themes of prediction and fallibility in psychoanalysis differ rather markedly from what is currently possible in the natural sciences. The problem of prediction in analytic therapy cannot be understood by making simple comparisons. To establish a valid prediction about the relation of processes which follow one upon the other with describable regularity is a goal common to all science. In psychoanalysis, the problem is a twofold one of making a warranted judgment and communicating it to the patient. And the many questions raised by this fact of communication are totally inapplicable in physics or chemistry. For example, it does not affect the activity of the oxygen molecule to assert that it

combines with two molecules of hydrogen under certain specifiable conditions to yield H_2O; nor does it have any effect on any
specific molecule whether it has been in that compound once or
a thousand times; nor does it make any difference who the ex-
perimenter happens to be, when he does the experiment or why
he does it, so long as he satisfies its required conditions. All of
these factors, however, are at the crux of the analytic situation:
because an assertion about a concatenation of events can affect
their future course through the action of suggestibility or the
counteraction of negative attitudes; because the history of an impersonal process is inexpendable to the consideration of its current function and future outcome; and it is by now common
knowledge that the personality of the analyst enters very much
into the analytic interaction.

Such imposing considerations make the style of derivation and
application of prediction in natural science comparatively useless in psychoanalysis. Even if a prediction is wrong, it can carry
such weight with the patient that he may attempt to produce the
conditions necessary for its realization—produce them, that is,
even when such conditions do not exist or contrary ones do exist.
It is an easily observed psychological fact that if one acts on the
assumption that certain things are true, the very activities based
on that assumption will in themselves eventually enstate the
truth of the assumption; and this holds true in man's relation to
both man and society, even though it is not always true in his
relation to nature.

The general pattern of scientific method is one and the same
in every discipline; the canons of scientific intelligibility are one
and the same in every field of empirical inquiry. A valid prediction is generally a warranted assertion about a series of events
which is based on descriptions of fact. Method is thus supremely
uniform in the human quest for reliable knowledge, even though
skills and usages vary from one subject matter to another. The
marked differences emerge in the specialized techniques of establishing and applying our knowledge.

The isolated and unrepeated event ordinarily has very limited interest for science. In psychoanalytic explorations of personality, however, what is least frequent may be most desirable. In a sense, our efforts in analytic therapy presuppose an inability to predict, for we gear our work toward the recognition of the emergence of the occasional irregularity in interpersonal processes. Certain operational cautions are therefore necessary in the study of repetitions. In fact, what is desired as a result of analytic therapy may never have occurred at all in the conscious memory of the patient. It can be an unrealized goal in interpersonal relations, wherefore the frequent defensive operations have to be analyzed in order to bring about the necessary conditions for its realization. If, then, a certain type of patient senses an extreme interest in frequent patterns of reaction, he can set out, consciously or unconsciously, to report and reproduce them with very little emotional involvement. Another type of patient will become overly anxious and find it impossible to report them altogether. Either way, the patient tries to satisfy at once the therapist's interest in such data and his own need to obstruct an intensive analysis of the defensive pattern. In this connection, it must be pointed out that patients will respond in accordance with their personal security needs no matter the therapeutic approach. Such transference responses to the study of personality disorders cannot of themselves rule out this approach to analytic therapy; besides, these side-effects often provide immediate clues to the specific ways in which the patient's anxieties are organized.

A warranted assertion about interpersonal processes is most useful for the enlargement of understanding after their occurrence. This may, at first blush, sound like an abuse of terms, but prediction is most useful in analytic therapy only after the patient has realized one concatenation of interpersonal processes or another in actual experience. The patient and his analyst can then begin to look into the operant factors which brought about the outcome it did in his life. They may then begin to look back at the various factors in past situations which produced the result they did. For after the event, the pressure of bias, prejudgment, influence or suggestion is minimal. And in this historical investigation the analyst can help to clarify these factors on the basis of the currently observed outcome which instigated this inquiry in the first place.

Insight may thus be a function of hindsight, but foresight is not solely a function of prediction even in this sense. It can also be a function of currently liberated energies, desires and impulses which may be directed at achieving a novel integration instead of duplicating the previous one which got him into trouble. This view does not, on the other hand, mean that the liberation of feelings is the therapeutic panacea; it is not a panacea because the mere liberation of feelings will only produce blinding chaos in the place of confusing crisis.

If to predict in advance of behavior, even when the canons of scientific inquiry point to a reliable and warranted prediction, can effect a weakening of the patient's prerogative in life, then it can also remove the analytic process from the domain of immediate experience, the well-spring of feeling, impulse and desire which infuse patterns of social behavior with vitality. This statement of the matter points up the connection between the generalized construct, but when such events are said to occur, they also can be studied in their significant effects. What is initially psychoanalytic art is geared. All absolutely induplicable events and all incommunicable feelings may be ruled out of the generalized construct, but such events occur, and when they do, they can also be studied in their significant effects. What is initially incommunicable and immutably private transcends the methods of science. Even though we later learn that it operates, prior to its emergence, beyond the universe of public discussion, it need not forever be consigned to its uniqueness within the realm of private experience. And to attempt a prediction in these circumstances introduces numerous intervening propositions which do not mean very much in themselves to a person in trouble. During consultations, they are experienced by the distraught patient as statistical manipulations, conceptual speculations, or at best as inferential operations which do not touch his emotional difficulties; and at worst, they are experienced as imposed metapsychological absolutes.

Although precise statistical frequencies cannot be established during therapeutic sessions, an elliptical use of the quantitative approach may be used, if one likes, to draw a general picture of how a person has managed to organize his life. It may also be used to establish the hypothetical dominance of certain goals of conduct and the lesser importance of others, or to assess the probable strength of each goal in relation to the others. But the standard procedures of natural science and animal psychology have three striking features which make them exceptionable from a psychoanalytic point of view. They are not intensive: the strength of an observable behavior is a simple function of its frequency, and any relation can be determined by a quantitative analysis of its observed appearance. They can merely be suggestive: the manner of introducing predictive hypotheses is decidedly more complicated in interpersonal relations than in physics or chemistry, for the authority of the therapist may overwhelm the patient to the extent that he will do what was "predicted"; the boundary line between prediction and suggestion, which is entirely irrelevant in natural science, is so difficult to maintain in social science. And they are definitely atomistic: the atomistic assumptions of statistical inference run counter to the principle of continuity underlying dynamic processes.

Let us look at these three general features a bit more closely. First of all, each person differs from every other one with respect to the organization, content and evaluation of his experience. There is no doubt that the method of psychoanalysis cannot be applied identically in every respect by any two people in any individual case, and every individual case is a case in itself. Consequently, it is extremely difficult to generalize about motives buttressing grossly similar behavior without neglecting significant personal aspects of these motives as uniquely organized in and through past experience. In fact, we often learn after a brief period of analysis that some habitual sequences of feeling may have been so repressed and so sharply defended against that they rarely appeared in open communication. When chiefly resistive and repressive patterns are finally expressed overtly, an exclusive use of hypotheses based on frequency analysis could mislead the observer and distort his picture of the basic constellation of attitudes and feelings. Furthermore, though quantitative measures are useful for some purposes, they fail to make certain aspects of emotions or meanings clear at all. For example, the article "the" occurs with much greater frequency in ordinary discussion than the noun "home," but this reveals nothing whatsoever about the differences in the psychological impact of these two words.

Secondly, predictive constructions which the patient produces about his interpersonal processes are considered most effective and useful. Instead of our analytic predictions, he needs a sense of significance in interpersonal experience. With it, he will be in a better position to understand how he got into his predicament, but we must remember that he still wants to decide on where he is going. Consequently, even if we can occasionally predict the eventual outcome of a given course of action, our ability to make the prediction does not entail our actually making it. Suggestion has been mentioned as one possible consequence. The counteraction of resistance, on the face of it an expression of the patient's right to live life as he sees it, has been mentioned as another. But even the superficial power of suggestion in the ordinary run of things should cause us to wonder what the patient really does when he carries out a suggestion of ours. For if the resolution were that simple, we would have to know why he could not see it on his own before analytic consultation. He may, in effect, be making it impossible for us to reach him and discover what he might like to suggest to himself under the circumstances.

Aside from the fact that current techniques of inquiry do not yield all of the data needed to make an accurate prediction about the behavior of the human organism, the above comments imply the final observation. Scientific techniques as developed in the natural sciences originally presupposed a mathematical and atomistic metaphysics. During the nineties, when Freud began to develop the psychoanalytic categories of explanation, he adapted the concepts of physics and physiology which presupposed the mathematico-mechanical nature of the human organism. He advanced "the conception that among the psychic functions there is something which should be differentiated (an amount of affect, a sum of excitation), something having all the attributes of quantity—although we possess no means of measuring it. . . . For the present it is justified by its utility in correlating and explaining diverse psychical conditions." [1] Today, we are still unable to obtain exact measurements of the increase, decrease, displacement and discharge of libidinal energy; and whether we will ever be able to do this is, for the present, an unanswerable question. However, if an alternative conceptual scheme can be "justified by its utility in correlating and explaining diverse psychical conditions," the use of Freud's quantitative conception is optional.

One of the most profound aspects of Freud's genius, it now appears, was his ability to investigate and describe psychodynamic processes in spite of the severe limitations imposed by this mathematico-mechanical frame of reference. For this metaphysical presupposition about the atomistic nature of man now has no significant therapeutic consequences. If it recommends itself to our attention, we are in no position to gather and apply the necessary information during consultations to secure mathematical validity; and of course if it does not, we simply do not need the information. None the less, the pursuit of this goal will only foster a mathematico-mechanical picture of man which does scant justice to his manifold potentialities and slights important characteristics of his dynamic psychological organization.

[1] S. Freud, "The Defence Neuro-Psychoses," *Collected Papers*, Volume I, London: 1924, p. 75.

---
chapter four

Transference: Positive and Negative

FREUD'S ANALYSIS of the case of Dora has a prominent place in the history of psychoanalytic therapy.[1] It was originally published in 1905, four years after the end of the analysis. It is the first case in which the new method of free association replaced his earlier therapies—both cathartic hypnosis with direct suggestion and concentration with interpretation of resistances. And one of his express reasons for publishing it was to illustrate the use of dream interpretation as an instrument of analytic therapy. In retrospect, however, the leading contribution of this case study is a finding which was only alluded to peripherally. It was a finding which eventually overshadowed all of his discoveries: the fact of transference in the therapeutic situation.[2]

From a second dream, reported two days before the end of treatment, Freud concluded that Dora unconsciously wanted to get revenge not only against Herr K., who had made advances to her, and her father, but—most important for its analytic implications—also against him. Transference was the term he used to identify her perception of the analyst as a substitute for both Herr K. and father; and her revenge was to discontinue in order to deprive him of a therapeutic success which he felt was almost within his reach. Though he did not get to the heart of Dora's transference distortions,[3] this failure paved the way to future

[1] Renewed interest in this case is evidenced by its current re-publication under separate cover as *The Case of Dora and Other Papers*, New York: 1952.

[2] S. Freud, "Fragment of an Analysis of a Case of Hysteria," *Collected Papers*, Volume III, London: 1925, pp. 139–144.

[3] Reference footnote 2, p. 141.

possibilities of therapeutic success—a not uncommon occurrence in the development of a science.

As far as Freud's earliest statement goes it is still unexceptionable: "What are transferences? They are new editions or facsimiles of the tendencies and phantasies which are aroused and made conscious during the progress of the analysis; but they have this peculiarity, which is characteristic for their species, that they replace some earlier person by the person of the physician. To put it another way; a whole series of psychological experiences are revived, not as belonging to the past, but as applying to the person of the physician at the present moment. Some of these transferences have a content which differs from that of their model in no respect whatever except for the substitution. These, then— to keep the same metaphor—are merely new impressions or reprints." [4] Though rather limited from theoretical and practical points of view, this statement holds the penetrating insight which, I think, made it possible for psychoanalysis to become what it is today. The developments of this momentous discovery during the last fifty years have resulted from voluminous experience and expansions in theory, but they stand as pale shadows in its powerful light.

Freud's therapeutic use of this formulation to describe Dora's distortions of him is open to question, however. He summed them up as a transference designed to get revenge against men— her father, Herr K. and himself. His construction of the concept of transference on the basis of Dora's analysis was a profound one, the more profound when seen against the background of the numerous hints and allusions in the discussion of her case which indicate that the dynamics of the current therapeutic situation were not taken into account.

Freud missed many factors in his current relationship with Dora, and in so doing, found himself in a helpless position when she set a date for finishing the analysis. Aside from this he had not as yet worked out his distinction between positive and negative transference; and the realistic as opposed to the distorted

[4] Reference footnote 2, p. 139.

side of the transference relationship had been overlooked. Nor
had he made the distinction between a negative transference distortion and a negative attitude toward the analyst based on what
he actually is, says or does. Unfortunately, it was also a technical
rule that positive transference was not to be touched analytically
until it had been transformed into resistance. And when this
transformation took place in the case of Dora, her analyst could
do nothing about it.

A few aspects of this case will be reviewed in order to point
up some of the other possibilities which are inherent in the data;
the importance of the current dynamic situation is emphasized
here as against historical and symbolic manipulation of what Dora
said. In the first place, she was not very interested in her analytic
therapy; this is evident in the many direct and indirect references
to her attitudes expressed about it. She entered treatment against
her will: Freud noted that "it was determined, *in spite of her
reluctance,* that she should come to me for treatment." [5] Or further on, "When I informed her of this condition (that she was
in love with Herr K.) she did not assent to it" [6]—while Freud
himself had little doubt about it as seen in his question on the
next page: "and how could a girl who was in love feel insulted
by a proposal which was made in a manner neither tactless nor
offensive?" [7] The possibility that she was not in love with Herr K.
might have been further considered. It might just as well have
been the frustrations she encountered in a loveless relationship
with her mother which were at the heart of the matter, since her
mother suffered from a "housewife's psychosis." Freud found it
easy "to substitute the sexual object of the moment (the penis)
for the original object (the nipple) or for the finger which did
duty for it later on." [8] This deft substitution by the creative use
of symbols is a tribute to his imaginative power, but it does not
eradicate our lingering doubts that Dora may have been seeking

[5] Reference footnote 2, p. 32, italics added.
[6] Reference footnote 2, p. 47.
[7] Reference footnote 2, p. 48.
[8] Reference footnote 2, p. 64.

the original object, the nipple and the maternal love it can represent; that she may have failed to obtain it even in her association with Frau K.; that perhaps Dora experienced Herr K.'s sexual advances to her as possible interferences in her relationship with Frau K.; and that she may actually have wanted to maintain some remnants of integrity in an inter-familial situation which certainly did not overflow with it.

Besides, there are numerous indications of power-struggles which went on between Freud and Dora, so that her leaving treatment may well have been a transference repetition to get revenge on her therapist. But it may also have been her realistic decision not to persist in power-struggles with a person who was presumably trying to help her with her problems. For instance, when they were working on the first dream, there was the following exchange at one point:

" 'Something occurs to me,' she said, 'but it cannot belong to the dream, for it is quite recent, whereas I have certainly had the dream before.'

" 'That makes no difference,' I replied, 'Start away! It will simply turn out to be the most recent thing that fits the dream.' " [9]

Now how Freud could have been so sure of this fact is difficult to comprehend; he had apparently not heard what it was that occurred to Dora: it might have been the color of the new wallpaper in the drawing room of her home, the latest performance of a Strauss waltz or any number of other fantastic, though not impossible, things. This response of Freud's suggests the temper of his inquiring attitude which did not give Dora a chance to try to make some sense out of her problem. Evidently, accidental and novel occurrences had no place in his therapeutic approach. If, for example, Dora reported that she had twisted her foot, there was a "requirement upon the fulfillment of which I had to insist. I am convinced that symptom of this kind can only arise where there is an infantile prototype." [10] Since he harbored this

[9] Reference footnote 2, p. 79; see p. 129 for other examples of it.
[10] Reference footnote 2, p. 125.

conviction with such firmness, she had to listen to his interpretation. But when she left treatment he considered it a transference
manifestation, not a response to antecedent convictions someone
else had about her experience which did not always accord with
her own.

Freud thought he was replacing Dora's father in her imagination: "She was even constantly comparing me with him consciously, and kept anxiously trying to make sure whether I was
being quite straight-forward with her, for her father 'always preferred secrecy and roundabout ways.' " [11] This might have been
an opening wedge to distinguish her experience of father from
her current relationship with Freud. Had he availed himself of
it, her initial reluctance to undertake psychoanalytic treatment
might have been mollified. And when her father reiterated his
disappointment in the treatment because Freud did not "talk"
Dora out of her knowledge about his affairs with Frau K., she
might not have discontinued treatment. Instead, she might have
continued in order to achieve a rather realistic revenge against
her father for having been devious, secretive and indirect.

And we come finally to Dora's leaving treatment just when
Freud thought successful termination was in sight. Was this necessarily "an unmistakable act of vengeance on her part?" [12] It can
be taken with equal cogency as a realistic response to a therapist
who failed to maintain a position of loyalty to his patient's best
interests as she saw them at that particular time. It was not seen
in connection with the cooling of her father's interest in psychoanalytic therapy when he discovered that Freud did not intend
to " 'talk' Dora out of her belief that there was something more
than a friendship between him and Frau K." [13] We know that
Dora was a reluctant patient whose therapeutic arrangements
were made by her father; also that he would not be satisfied with
Dora's retaining her beliefs about his affairs with Frau K.; but
we do not know, from Freud's report, what happened in these

11 Reference footnote 2, p. 141.
12 Reference footnote 2, p. 131.
13 Reference footnote 2, p. 131.

various relationships during the treatment, especially her father's reactions to its progress.

Dora's unplanned termination may have been "an unmistakable act of vengeance" against Freud on a quite realistic basis in order to regain some measure of her self-esteem; its distorted and self-destructive quality may have been her desire to get revenge against father who brought her for analytic therapy against her will. By this act of denying herself the possibilities of further analysis, she may have gained revenge against both of them for quite different reasons.

But hindsight is always easier than foresight. Today, even though this remains an undecidable issue, it is decidedly clear that the data in the case are not exempt from further examination. At the present stage of psychoanalytic development, however, it makes little difference that Freud's description of Dora's transference distortions is open to serious question because he missed the significance of current factors in the therapeutic relationship. The fact that Freud was able to formulate his first psychoanalytic statement of the transference phenomenon in this case is not really affected by the actual course of the analysis of Dora's transference manifestations. It matters little that he had not "mastered" the finer structure of her interpersonal involvements. The salient fact is that his discovery of transference in the therapeutic situation was first published in this case.

In 1918 Freud wrote that when transference was positive, it conferred authority upon the analyst because it indicated faith in the analyst's findings and views; the analyst, he thought, would not even be listened to without this sort of transference.[14] However, this view overestimates the value and need for positive transference in analytic therapy. It also prevented him from inspecting the negative attitudes, distorted or real, which were clothed in the positive transference. This is a very revealing statement, for it opens to question all findings with which the patient concurred during a positive transference and all views which he

14 S. Freud, *A General Introduction to Psychoanalysis*, Garden City: 1943, p. 387.

accepted because of the analyst's authority. But it misses the factual mark. The strongest faith in the analyst's findings derives from the patient's own review of these findings in the light of his own understanding, and with sufficient contact—that is, so long as a negative transference does not cause the discontinuation of treatment, it may be possible to demonstrate to the patient that his negative transference, when it is a composite of distortions, interferes with his perceptions of the analyst.

In his analysis of Dora Freud had already begun grappling with this problem. It is interesting to note an opinion he had presented in 1905 that is very close to the contemporary one: "Transference, which seems ordained to be the greatest obstacle to psychoanalysis, becomes its most powerful ally, if its presence can be detected each time and explained to the patient." [15] What happened to this idea during the intervening years is difficult to trace in his writings. Why he later changed his mind and decided that positive transference distortions were not to be touched until they became resistance is not at all clear unless we make the inference that he had changed his mind about their role in the interim. He may have decided that it was better to capitalize on a positive transference as long as one could get something done rather than upset the equilibrium, though he also knew in advance that it would be transformed into resistance or negative transference and the equilibrium would be upset anyway. Yet Freud's idea that transference distortions be detected each time and explained to the patient, though he had suffered a therapeutic failure in this case, still seems to be valid. For if an analyst has deaf ears to the first notes of transference distortion, he will allow them to become crescendo. They can take him unawares in this way, and do more harm in placing him in the position of not being able to analyze it in full emotional force than good because the patient will not have had any gradual introduction to the understanding of its manifestations.

Most analysts are by now accustomed to the experience of surprise, and were this the sole outcome, little more would need to

15 Reference footnote 2, p. 141.

be said about it. But the patient will, in this circumstance, go sailing on the crest of a transference experience without knowing what it is all about. It is most helpful to have some sort of organized picture of the patient's personality before a transference distortion gets into full swing. It must make some sort of interpersonal sense to the analyst before it wells up, and this is why he should begin his probings at its earliest manifestations. When this has not been worked out, both the analyst and the patient are more or less in the dark during the experience. Another factor to be considered in this connection is the fruitless expenditure of effort and time and money which the patient hopefully makes with the expectation of acquiring understanding of his distortions. For if the analyst is at sea, the patient in the throes of a transference distortion is not only also at sea; he has unnecessarily undergone an experience of anxiety of unknown proportions.

This does not of course mean that the unfolding of a transference distortion can in any way be hindered if it has to unfold; if it has to, it will. Besides such distortions in perception must be felt, and they must be gone through, if an analysis of their sources and functions are to have meaning. Once the analyst has crucial working clues about the patient's life, he follows the lead of the patient's communications. The purpose of following this unfolding of transference distortions is not to look for positive transferences in order to guide suggestibility or test reality; the purpose is that the patient experience them profoundly so that he will always be able to refer to them when he gets hazy about his potential for distorting perceptions. In fact, he can often use the recall of such experiences during analysis as a focus about which to organize his new knowledge about himself.

This is a conceptualization of what happens when an analysis of transference distortion is underway. Empirically, it does not always work in this way because the analyst cannot manage all of the variables and does not always know in advance whether any specific defense is the most significant one. After a segment of analysis is done, he just has to wait and see no matter how successfully he may feel the transference distortion has been analyzed. Nor is it always possible to obtain sufficient clues before a transference experience gets started. Again, he may just have to wait and be prepared for the unexpected to occur without becoming impatient and anticipating what will happen. He listens with the third ear, as the current vogue has it; the import of this metaphor is that he is no longer listening to the patient's reports because he can no longer keep abreast of them. When he listens with the third ear, he has distracted his attention from what the patient is presently saying and has begun to listen to his own reactions to what is going on. And as this is communicated—usually non-verbally—to the patient, it is often found that the patient has also begun to listen to himself. There are occasions when the analyst has to drift with the theme or mood of the session and see what will occur to himself and the patient.

Ideally, the analysis of transference takes place throughout the psychotherapeutic process. As soon as there is sufficient indication to question the meaning of a certain bit of distorted behavior, then questioning is appropriate. Freud recognized that the transference existed in the patient from the very beginning of analytic therapy.[16] But he also noted that nothing is seen of it,[16] and this is highly dubious. Alertness even to characteristic mannerisms of speech or to typical ways of opening and closing sessions, for example, can disclose significant facts. One need not go along with the apparently favorable effects of the therapeutic work and wait until it becomes reoriented into a defensive process before paying serious attention to it.

In Freud's last view of this matter transference distortions that were, in the analyst's judgment, positive and favorable to the work were actually allowed to avalanche, and the analyst, perhaps unwittingly but none the less effectively, fostered their transformation into resistance. In one place he had ascribed the following characteristics to positive transference: docility, acceptance of analytic explanations, remarkable comprehension and

16 Reference footnote 14, pp. 384–385. This assertion, that nothing is seen of it, supports the opinion, incidentally, that Freud ordinarily did not treat positive transference as a distortion at all—not, at least, until it became transformed into a negative one.

a high degree of intelligence.[17] He proceeded to describe the disappearance of these qualities when transference-love emerged. Today, the first two would ordinarily require some sort of inquiry from the very outset. If the patient showed an all too ready acceptance of analytic explanations, the therapist would look into her docility. For if her comprehension were so rapid and remarkable, he would wonder why she had not arrived at these explanations on her own prior to psychoanalytic consultation; and since she had a high degree of intelligence, she must also have noted these facts even if she could not do much about understanding them.

In his discussion of transference-love Freud also noted that it "can express itself in less tender feelings" [18] than affection but he did not pursue this aspect of it. And this hostile and manipulative side of transference-love has as its purpose to avoid the feelings of hopelessness about really finding someone who can love and be loved in return. Also noteworthy in this connection is the patient who seeks to deny her objectionable qualities, more often imagined than real, by indirectly and unconsciously evoking such denials from the analyst and thereby ensuring her defenses against her unconscious feelings about herself. It is frequently observed that patients who have seductive fantasies do not really hope to seduce the analyst; in fact, their hopes are founded on the desire to avoid the discovery of their sexual anxieties. The implicit rationalization seems to be that no one would suspect the presence of sexual fears or fears of personal intimacy if such unfettered fantasies could be expressed.

Simply put, the role of anxiety is clear and graphic. It antecedes and touches off the fantastic distortions, while the content of the fantasies, in transference-love as in other gross distortions, provides significant clues to the factors initiating anxiety. The mere repetition of professions of love does not add such to the psychological data; it does emphasize, however, that the patient is probably involved with her analyst in an anxious and defensive

[17] S. Freud, "Observations on Transference-Love," *Collected Papers*, Volume II, London: 1924, p. 381.

[18] Reference footnote 17, p. 379 fn.

way. Her aim is generally to get reassurance about her worthiness
and acceptability; its source is often an historically grounded fear
of being manipulated and so, in view of the realistic character of
the therapeutic relationship, transference-love serves to keep the
analyst at a distance. The interesting thing about the appearance
of this kind of transference is that it can occasionally produce the
very condition it seeks to avoid: she may become unacceptable
as an analytic patient. For if the analyst were to reciprocate his
patient's feelings and fall in love with her, he would automatically
disqualify himself from continuing the analysis.

The interweaving of psychological processes, genetically as well
as functionally, is much more complex, and it points up the need
to inquire after the manifestations of transference as soon as they
are evident. The realistic structure of the therapeutic relationship indicates such an approach: analytic consultations are ordinarily undertaken because the patient needs help and the analyst is able to provide it. Hence the need for tactful confrontation
of transference-love immediately and directly, lest its current
functions within the analytic situation go unnoticed and its unconscious expectations actually come into being. If transference-
love goes unnoticed, it camouflages this structure and tends to
undermine it.

This constellation of processes may also be observed in other
expressions of transference distortion. For example, if a patient's
pronounced passive dependency has incurred the abuse of others
once he became involved in such a relationship—and he later
recognized this abuse for what it was and reacted to it in a negative and hostile way, then this principle that the analyst not
trouble himself with passive dependency, so long as the patient
did what he was supposed to do and developed a positive transference, would actually foster the ensuing hostility. When, under
these circumstances, the transference toward the analyst becomes
negative and hostile, it does not necessarily mean that he has
been put in the place of one or the other of the patient's parents. It often means that this negativism and hostility have occurred just because the analyst attempted to influence and guide

the patient's suggestibility without his awareness and express accord. Freud made the mistaken observation that the achievement of an affectionate positive transference had positive therapeutic value, while the need for active analysis only arose with the emergence of obstacles to the suggestive powers of the analyst. Yet the fact of the matter seems to be that passive dependency is nurtured in the soil of repressed hostility, for no self-respecting person can permit others to make his decisions for him without recognizing the discrepancy between his responsibility to himself and the restrictions which others have imposed on that responsibility. To allow an apparently positive transference to develop without attempts at therapeutic intervention conveys to the patient that the analyst is but another in a series of individuals in his life who want to run things for him. Freud's observation hits snags of another sort when confronted with that type of aggressive dependency which does not allow a positive transference to evolve in a clear state anyway. The apparently disowned or denied dependency, which is the so-called positive transference again, requires paramount attention, since the aggressivity in the presenting picture is, by its intensity, an unusually reliable index of the concomitant dependency that is evident in its denial.

Freud's sharp distinction between positive and negative transference is misleading. It can even obscure the essentially psychoanalytic task of working with distorted aspects of perception. The trouble with classifying transference into positive and negative types is, moreover, that this classification does not take into account the vast differences of nuance and shading in this range. Every transference manifestation is a specific distortion, and the decision about its positive or negative quality usually depends on how the analyst happens to judge it. But the patient does not really need any such judgment on the character of his transference distortions. Though the analyst may derive some security from his ability to say at least something about the distortion, these terms are at best superfluous. The patient needs to define and study his distortions genetically and functionally in order to

resolve them. And it really does not increase the understanding
of either the analyst or the patient to label them positive or negative from the analyst's perspective. These terms convey nothing
of the singular character of any specific difficulty as it is organized and functioning in the patient's life. Furthermore, to call it
positive or negative may imply that an analyst can work with a
positive transference but cannot work with a negative one. But
this implication is false because no matter the quality or content
of the distortion, it has to be seen as an obstacle to analysis and
treated as such. Besides, there are occasions when positive transference may contain a much more complicated distortion and a
negative attitude may be a relatively clear perception.

This classification of transferences had as a corollary the idea
that affect constituted the transference distortion; for it was affect alone that Freud, in following the "electric current" conception of psychic energy, considered positive or negative. But a
transference manifestation is not merely a psychic affect toward
specific personality characteristics of the analyst. It is a distorted
concretion of all past experiences which unfold in the perception
of these characteristics. It is the total personality in distorted reaction. No transference distortion presents itself simply or directly in the affective mode, and the analytic focus of interest is
not limited to its affective traits. It presents no consistent picture
of being solely or simply positive or negative. It is a complex experience which we have to unravel and follow into past experiences and future expectancies.

A dynamic and changing constellation of feelings and attitudes
emerges when we take this course. Transference distortions would
lose their vital and compelling quality if one or another of these
factors in the total constellation were abstracted to the exclusion
of the others and were thought to set the dominant theme of the
total constellation. And they would certainly lose their personal
meaning if this abstracted factor were reduced entirely to its affective tone, positive or negative; for it is humanly impossible to
study any feeling or affective tone in total abstraction from
thought or context. Theoretically, if the analyst is competent and

interested and the patient capable and motivated, the analysis of any distorted concretion of past experience and future expectation would lead in all directions like the spokes of a wheel to past interpersonal involvements with different people. This is not usually necessary for therapeutic purposes, because the most effective therapeutic efforts are those which point up "here and now" experiences.

Practically speaking, we follow one factor rather than others because its frequency, compulsion or urgency is prominent in the context of a particular therapeutic problem; or because this one factor may point in a more constructive direction than another. But this sort of selective analysis does not reduce the total constellation to its affective quality or to the affective quality of any of its constituent factors. It does not require that we dichotomize transference manifestations and place them in one of two rubrics. Though chiefly concerned with function, it goes to the content of the constellation, finds some factors more significant than others for the problem at hand, and follows them up without prejudging the possible worth of the other factors which have been left behind. For these may turn out to be of overriding importance at some future date when the context of the problem becomes transformed. Thus we often have to return to this complex distortion to pick up other elements which have begun to loom larger because of the way the problem is shaping up or because new problems have appeared which have been precipitated or made clearer by these formerly unessential factors.

Since World War II there has been a revival of interest in techniques of brief psychotherapy. Numerous variations of these methods of guiding positive transference and hypnosis have, of course, been among them. This interest has been fostered by occasional striking results in cases of a traumatic sort; these cases are usually typified by rather recent and severe environmental dislocations. The dynamic psychological conditions to which these short-term techniques have proved applicable do not differ significantly from those in which Freud discovered the utility of positive transference. None has been able to disregard this trans-

ference factor either theoretically or therapeutically. Especially
where unconscious dependency is marked do these positive transferences sustain themselves in and through distorted expectations
from powerful people in authority as prototypes of important
figures in past experience.

The analysis of these distorted figures can only take place, according to current conceptions and techniques, in the analysis of
the total personality, taking the career-line of the individual as
its basis for investigation into the constituents of his character
structure. Out of such an investigation there emerge certain recurrent patterns of interaction which provide the grist for the
continued mill of disturbance. Rioch has demonstrated the pitfalls of suggestion, exhortations and pontifical pronouncements
by carefully delineating the manner in which the basis of later
transference manifestations has usually been laid in childhood by
the mothering one's injunctions and cajolery.[19]

Under certain exigent circumstances the therapist may have no
alternative to a short-term course of treatment. The assumption
is that if the patient has worked through some central distortion
in one area of his life, imaginative resources will be freed to deal
with distortions in other areas of his life. The skill of the therapist lies in his ability to size up what is actually going on in the
patient's life and how successfully the presenting difficulties have
been resolved. Nevertheless, he must ultimately take the patient's
report as final. There is no joint validation of the evidence, since
the short-term therapist is limited by the memory and communicational screen of the patient which cannot be inquired after
since it was initially ruled out by the limited objectives of the
therapeutic course.

[19] J. Rioch, "The Transference Phenomenon in Psychoanalytic Therapy,"
Psychiatry VI (1943), pp. 147–156.

chapter five

Suggestion in the Shape
of Transference

TO READ FREUD'S THEORY of transference sympathetically, it is necessary to make a conscious effort to get into his hypnotic and authoritarian frame of reference. For when he rediscovered suggestion in the shape of transference, he did not mean what we mean by transference today. This difference in meaning may be gleaned from his rather specifically described method of working with transference suggestion in a frame of reference which was firmly rooted in hypnotic psychotherapy. Many of his statements appear to be inconsistent from our current vantage point, but in his system of thought they are consistent. Despite this logical consideration, however, neither his analytic method nor his frame of reference does justice to current clinical observations. By not reading his ideas into current conceptions of psychoanalytic therapy, we may avoid these inconsistencies. So, looking backward, with our increasing clarity about transference distortion, we find it difficult to use his conceptual scheme in order to help a patient find his way to freedom of expression and power to act.

One of Freud's major problems in the *Introductory Lectures* was to differentiate transference analysis from direct suggestion. In one place he held that the late nineteenth-century theories of suggestibility described nothing but the tendency to transference. He objected to Bernheim's views solely on the ground that Bernheim could not explain the rise and function of the suggestive process because its relationship to the libido was not recognized.[1] This disagreement with Bernheim actually posed the problem of

[1] S. Freud, *A General Introduction to Psychoanalysis,* Garden City: 1943, p. 387.

67

the nature of transference; it did not resolve anything. With equal cogency it might be said that Freud never differentiated syntaxic from parataxic suggestion because he was blinded by his belief in the dependence of suggestibility on the functioning of the libido. That he recognized the shortcomings of his statement of the issue is clearly evident from the fact that he devoted a large part of the following lecture—the twentieth-eighth—to it. I will reviews its highlights, for it clearly demonstrates that his method of transference analysis was a suggestive technique designed to cure symptoms just like his earlier therapeutic techniques. And his failure to progress beyond this goal of treatment indicates that he had never freed himself from the influences of his early training in hypnosis and direct suggestion.

When suggestion was aimed directly against the symptoms, a struggle arose, as Freud saw it, between the therapist's authority and the underlying motives of the neurosis.[2] However, the process of recovery in analytic treatment was also described in terms of a struggle between the analyst's authority and the motives underlying the patient's problem: the important phase of the analysis was to be carried through by creating new editions of those early conflicts in the transference relationship; the patient would try to behave as he originally did, while the analyst utilized every available resource he had to bring about another resolution. The analysis of transference, to repeat, was the field on which the crucial battles were waged.[3] Apparently, the difference between direct suggestion and suggestion in the shape of transference was that in the latter the analyst secured a better position from which to make his direct suggestion; and he now aimed his suggestions more purposefully at the resistances instead of at one or another facet of the conflict. This difference was chiefly a procedural one. In the former, suggestion was consciously directed at the content of the conflict, while in the latter, it was directed at its structure and process, the content being allowed to enter awareness to be resolved in its own terms as an ordinary psychological conflict.

[2] Reference footnote 1, p. 390.
[3] Reference footnote 1, p. 395.

The change was thus a change in the purpose to which suggestion was put. As in the early *Studies in Hysteria,* it was still used to struggle with the patient, and the special significance of the new technique was that Freud could now direct his efforts more accurately and center his suggestions squarely on resistance in their new and forceful form, the transference phenomenon. This innovation was in itself a revolutionary one. Instead of entering the conflictual struggle of the patient, the battlefield was moved over to the psychological resistances and limitations that fed into the conflict—but battlefield it remained; and removing the resistances to repression in order to recover lost memories remained the goal of both hypnotic psychotherapy and psychoanalysis.

This point is further sharpened by comments such as these: In one place, Freud wrote that it now became possible for the analyst to use his powers of suggestion in entirely new ways; he could control the suggestive process; and in so far as the patient was open to its influence, his suggestibility was guided by the analyst.[4] On the next page he noted that the resolution of the transference relationship marked the end of the analysis, but this could not be accomplished without the help of suggestion in overcoming resistances.[5] And further on, he relied on suggestion very explicitly as the analyst's means of bringing the patient's distorted object-relations into awareness where they could be worked out as an ordinary psychological problem.[6]

If we turn to Freud's last work, *An Outline of Psychoanalysis,* there is no modification of this construction to be found. He wrote in one place, "However much the analyst may be tempted to act as teacher, model and ideal to other people and to make men in his own image, he should not forget that that is not his task in the analytic relationship. . . He will only be repeating one of the mistakes of the parents, when they crushed their child's independence, and he will be replacing one kind of dependence by another. In his attempts at improving and educat-

[4] Reference footnote 1, p. 393.
[5] Reference footnote 1, p. 394.
[6] Reference footnote 1, p. 395.

ing the patient the analyst must respect his individuality." [7] And so far as contemporary work in transference analysis is concerned, this view of the matter is unimpeachable. But it was written after the following: "This transference is ambivalent: it comprises positive and affectionate as well as negative and hostile attitudes towards the analyst, who, as a rule, is put in the place of one or other of the patient's parents, his father or his mother. So long as it is positive it serves us admirably." [8] Yet two pages later we read, "Therapeutic successes that take place under the sway of the positive transference are under suspicion of being of a *suggestive* nature." [9] And nine pages later: "We serve the patient in various functions as an authority and a substitute for his parents, as a teacher and educator" [10]—and this without any caution to analyze positive transference.

Now both of these views cannot recommend themselves equally for our support. Either positive transference serves us admirably, in which case its therapeutic successes are under no suspicion at all; or its therapeutic successes may be suspected of being suggestive in nature, in which case it does not serve us admirably at all. This ambiguity may be due to the fact that Freud never distinguished between parataxic and syntaxic suggestion—because therapeutic successes which occur during positive transference are indeed of a suggestive nature. And to mention in passing a point to which I will return: When Freud allowed positive transference to serve him admirably, the ensuing negative and hostile transference need not have been seen as necessarily and solely connected with attitudes toward parents during the oedipal period. The possibility has to be considered that the negative and hostile transference was actually directed against the analyst for having allowed the patient's parataxic suggestibility to serve his therapeutic efforts instead of analyzing it when he had sufficient evidence for its existence. Or, if the so-called negative transfer-

---

[7] S. Freud, *An Outline of Psychoanalysis,* New York: 1949, p. 67
[8] Reference footnote 7, p. 66.
[9] Reference footnote 7, p. 68–69.
[10] Reference footnote 7, p. 77.

ence never clearly emerged in any given case, it might never have to be looked for just because its opposite had served the analyst's purposes admirably.

In Freud's day suggestion was generally taken in a simple way: one made the suggestion and the recipient performed what it contained.[11] Dynamic considerations had hardly received any consideration at the turn of the century, and suggestion was largely used as a suppressive agency. It was with his discovery of neurotic defenses, among other things, that Freud decided that he had to go it alone. The courageous imagination required to have given up the techniques of hypnosis and direct suggestion at that time is difficult for us to evaluate from our vantage point. The new concept of suggestion in the form of transference was certainly a step forward when seen against the backdrop of the ideas of his predecessors and contemporaries. Yet, from our current perspective, it is also possible to note that the virus of hypnotic suggestion and its authoritarian matrix were not entirely expunged from his method of transference analysis. In fact, there were two incompatible strains in his therapeutic conceptions: an analytic technique which was the antithesis of the hypnotic goal and a hypnotic goal which was the antithesis of analytic technique. In the case of Dora, he had described the inutility of the earlier techniques that were totally inadequate for dealing with "the finer structure of a neurosis";[12] the other step, to surrender the aims and goals of those techniques, was not given to him to take.

To state this matter a bit more schematically: The increasingly important consideration of the finer structure of a neurosis differed from the overwhelming concern with symptoms; the technique of free association differed from that of prohibition, reassurance or counter ideas; but the fact of suggestion was common to both the earlier and the later points of view, and just how transference suggestion in analytic therapy was intrinsically dif-

11 W. James, *Principles of Psychology*, Volume II, New York: 1890, Chapter XXVII.

12 S. Freud, "A Fragment of an Analysis of a Case of Hysteria," *Collected Papers*, Volume III, London: 1925, p. 19.

ferent from suggestion in an hypnotic state was never made clear.
Since Freud retained his idea that resistance was developed solely
to repress early memories, there could not have been any fundamental points of difference between hypnotic suggestion and
transference suggestion. If we were to hold fast to his own view
of the matter—that the change in procedure was made because
certain patients simply were not hypnotizable, we would be left
with the idea that his mode of operation did not change. And
since the therapeutic aims remained identical throughout, we
may conclude that all procedural changes were made the better
to achieve those very aims.

This problem cannot be resolved by translating it into a theoretical problem and simply asserting that suggestibility be understood in terms of libidinal development. The therapeutic meaning
and utility of suggestion require far more than apriori definition to be made intelligible. They are to be found in what Freud
did with it. And he said he did one thing: overcame the inner
resistances of the patient against returning to the past in order
to face again and work through a childhood trauma with the help
of suggestion; his chief aim was to recover lost memories. It was
irrelevant that his authoritarian mode of suggestion relied on the
patient's unconscious dependencies during the so-called positive
transference; and he did not, to my knowledge, consider this
question in any of his writings. The recovery of lost memories
was a kind of end-in-itself and all means which could be successfully employed on "the battlefield of transference" to realize
it were fair and warranted; how this end was realized during the
transference experience was less important to him than that it
be realized.

That the recall of the repressed would turn the therapeutic
trick was, in itself, a certain and foregone conclusion. His therapeutic goal, once set for him by hypnotherapy, apparently maintained the status of a supreme goal; and like all supreme goals,
no matter how pursued, its attainment would yield the desired
therapeutic rewards. This being the case, it was probably an

exciting event for Freud to have discovered that he had never entirely quit his first psychotherapeutic discipline, but that he had only modified its procedures to rediscover suggestion again in the form of transference. So far as he was concerned, the circle was completed.

Freud was well aware of this fact. In the final statement of his analytic conceptions of therapy he saw the difference between his earlier and later procedures as follows: Hypnotic psychotherapy employed suggestion to prohibit the persistence of the symptoms; in so doing, it actually reinforced the repression without any change in the processes which conditioned the formation of the symptoms. Analytic therapy, on the other hand, struck at the roots of the neurosis and tackled the conflicts from which the symptoms developed; yet it also used suggestion to affect the eventual course of the basic conflicts.[13] But was this not also the aim of Breuer's cathartic technique? Freud did not change the purpose of suggestive interventions when he changed from the cathartic technique to the methods of concentration and free association. Nor did he redefine it as a leading principle when he carried it over into psychoanalytic therapy. To be sure, it was used at a different level of awareness in transference analysis than in hypnosis. Instead of going directly to the roots of the symptoms under a hypnotic trance, the symptoms were now sought out indirectly by the interpretation of transference resistance. But he had not considered the possibility that transference suggestion could have as distorted a base as hypnotic suggestion whether directed at overt manifestations of conflict or at its underlying determinants. And he could not take this step because he had no distinction between syntaxic and parataxic suggestion.

A word about this choice of terminology may be helpful at this point. It was motivated by the observation that both distorted and non-distorted attitudes possess rational factors in addition to the many irrational factors involved. Sullivan's notions of para-

[13] Reference footnote 1, p. 392.

taxic and syntaxic [14] are well suited to set off this difference because, unlike terms like rational and irrational, they do not
stress the presence or absence of intelligence as such but focus
instead on the nature of the current perception, on whether its
referents are current contexts or whether contexts of past experience intrude and dominate it. Even the most parataxic attitude
requires some measure of intelligence for its enactment and the
most syntaxic suggestion requires some measure of feeling for it
to take hold in life. Also worthy of note in this connection is the
desirability of providing a conceptual ground for such processes
as unconscious intellectual defenses which, though irrational,
certainly employ intelligence to an uncanny degree. As distinctions among interpersonal processes, parataxic and syntaxic cannot be isolated from each other; they are compresent and compenetrating in life-experience, the problem in therapy being to
separate the wheat from the chaff. The syntaxic mode represents
an ideal limit which is easiest to define negatively as the increasing absence of parataxic factors. The parataxic mode, on the
other hand, refers to the automatic introduction of feelings and
attitudes into contexts of experience where they have no function discernible in terms of the objective conditions. This notion
of parataxic experience marks an advancement in descriptive
terminology because it stresses the fact that transference distortions emerge within "me-you" patterns of communication and
relatedness; that they originally grew out of "me-you" patterns
and recur in them; and that those which we study do not persist in any individual and mentalistic repository such as the Collective Unconscious or the Systematic Unconscious.

What is syntaxic suggestion? In what ways are we concerned
with it in our therapy? How do we employ it? And what does
it mean in relation to the analysis of transference? The fact is
that suggestions, conscious and unconscious, are made all of the

14 H. S. Sullivan, *Conceptions of Modern Psychiatry*, Washington, D.C.:
1947, p. 45; also P. Mullahy, *Oedipus: Myth and Complex*, New York: 1948,
pp. 286–291 and C. Thompson, *Psychoanalysis: Evolution and Development*,
New York: 1950, p. 216.

time in therapeutic work. For instance, we often focus on a character trait as the problem to be investigated; or we do not always respond to a patient's reaction which we consider distorted; occasionally, we also communicate to our patients by word or gesture our opinion of the probable outcome of a given course of action. Such suggestions may be necessary and should be made without hesitation when indicated; but they do not constitute analysis.

Suggestion is syntaxic or parataxic depending not only on the intent and frame of reference from which it is made but also on the frame of reference in which it is received. During the so-called positive transference, suggestions would find unconscious support in the covert dependency problems of the patient; indeed during any transference process, whatever its emotional quality in the analyst's judgment, suggestions are seen and taken distortedly by the patient. Were the patient in the throes of any sort of transference distortion of the analyst, it would follow, moreover, that the chief force of the suggestion would be parataxic, regardless of the attitudinal context from which it was extended. Thus the syntaxicity of a suggestion depends on the psychological condition of the participants—on whether the therapist has unresolved authority needs and whether the patient's parataxic dependencies are resolved or are in the center of the therapeutic situation.

The therapeutic expectation that authoritative suggestions will be effective is based on the proposition that psychological processes are discrete, separate and isolable. But no perception, whether or not it is congruent with current facts, can be maintained in isolation; it is organized into continuous and interdependent patterns extending over wide areas of beliefs and experiences. This matrix of belief and experience from which single processes arise may be called the frame of reference or the backdrop against which they occur; it is the "finer structure of the neurosis" to which Freud referred in his case of Dora. This frame of reference cannot be suggested away. Such suggestion would in fact be parataxic on the part of the analyst because it

would entail psychological powers he does not possess. Most
peripheral processes usually persist in one frame of reference as
easily as in another. They can readily be repatterned in a new
form of expression so that authoritative suggestion will become
a constant crutch in order to effect such shifts in peripheral function. For the specific idea, opinion, defense or symptom is of less
therapeutic significance than the frame of reference in which it
operates.

We know that a well timed suggestion by the analyst may effect transient shifts of opinion or a temporary removal of symptoms. However, if it is enforced by the unconscious authority of
the analyst or the unconscious dependency of the patient, as it
usually is, then we must assume that the situation has remained
as ambiguous and as fluid as it was before—this opinion or symptom or whatever psychological process being subject to change
again. Such suggestion is effective as a therapeutic technique
when it has a clear field of unconscious dependency and ignorance in which to operate. If distortions are rectified by simply
seeking out authoritative judgments about the nature of the situation and how it is to be perceived, an unsatisfactory condition
would be created in which the authority would continually need
to be consulted to make such judgments. If they are singled out
as facts to be investigated, they may be clarified by being ignored
as such and studied genetically and functionally as symptomatic
offshoots of other interpersonal experiences. The skilled analysis
of transference stops short of suggestions which depend for their
effectiveness on distorted dependency—not the casual suggestions
and comments about everyday affairs which humans are bound
to make but those that are intended to have a therapeutic outcome.

A suggestion is really the posing of an alternative to the presented possibilities or the reinforcing of a desired possibility at
any particular point in a problem-solving situation. Valid changes
in judgment ordinarily occur because the material to be judged
is seen in a different perspective; some aspect or some factor acquires a new context and, as a consequence, acquires another

meaning. Where a person is incapable of clear perception, suggestion can only be parataxic. It follows of course that changes in judgment do not occur—nor do suggestions succeed for that matter—where the perceived field is stable and unambiguous. Suggestion, syntaxic or parataxic, can operate only when the matters under consideration are susceptible to more than one meaning, outcome or course of action. If the analyst makes a suggestion which he considers to be a valid one, then he has no especially personal stake in its being carried out; it has the same merit as the suggestion of the butcher, the baker or the candlestick maker—that is, the patient may accept it or reject it on its own merits irrespective of the position of the analyst. Since the authority of scientific intelligence is impersonal, the compelling force of the analyst's comments and inferences is not vested in the authority of his person or position. And while it rests on the authority of psychoanalytic knowledge which has been derived from wide technical experience, the proof of the pudding, so far as the patient is concerned, is still in the eating. In the psychoanalytic situation where channels of communication are unfettered by dogma and where integrations of the participants are unhampered by conventional habits of communication, open inquiry will eventually yield public truth.

Instead of a procedure that uses suggestion to change the outcome of conflicts, our therapeutic goal is set by a procedure which goes after the characteristic sources of conflict which make the employment of suggestion necessary in the first place. The goal is to analyze transference distortions which limit the patient's syntaxic suggestibility—a readiness to perceive his current life-situations as they occur without interferences from past experience, a willingness to hear alternative courses of action in that current situation, and an ability to decide on the valid merits of the case without looking for approval or disapproval to limit the encroachments of anxiety. If perception be considered an organized act which is warranted by specific occurrences in one's life-situation, then distortions in perception may be said to change when there are changes in the organization of the psychological factors in that situation. This is of course an oversimplified statement which will have to be expanded in the next chapter.

The aim of analysis is not to suggest alternative ways of perceiving an ambiguous and unstable situation. It is not to exploit the analyst's position of authority as a magical source of truth for patients when they are confused and do not know what to do. The analytic task is to inquire why other alternatives do not suggest themselves to the patient, what blocks his capacity for insight and foresight into the ambiguous and unstable, and why he seeks suggestions to clarify his difficulties rather than to clarify his need for suggestions. The aim of constructive analysis is definitely not reeducation. Its goal is to find, by inquiring into transference distortions, what has blocked the patient's way to whatever reeducational sources he wishes in order to pursue his goals. Patients do not ordinarily consult an analyst in order to be reeducated, and analysts do not describe their services as being those of a reeducator. Thus, to work through to the point where the patient is open to syntaxic suggestion is one thing; to get him to the point where he is open to any specific types of suggestion is quite another thing, and if the latter were the aim of analysis, it would destroy analysis as a unique form of psychotherapy. The patient's capacity to make syntaxic decisions may enable him to choose between alternatives without the intervention of parataxic distortions of the analyst and others—and this is the condition which analysis aims to bring about.

It was Freud's dim view of achieving therapeutic results through the analysis of negative transference which influenced him to conclude his last major discussion of the transference phenomenon on the note that he had given up hypnosis only to rediscover suggestion again in the shape of transference.[15] During the transference experience, however, even during the so-called positive transference, patients are least accessible to syntaxic sug-

[15] Reference footnote 1, p. 388. This statement of his hypnotic conception of transference confirms the thesis that he never really explored the magnitude of his original discovery in his analysis of Dora.

gestion. Positive or negative transferences usually convey distortions of commonly perceived relationships and qualities; to accept its manifestations at face value is to accept a falsehood. The therapeutic work is deflected from its course by the repressed experiences which have not as yet been disclosed and analyzed. As a result, the attendant anxieties are aroused and they introduce impassable barriers to the continuance of open two-way communication. When direct or indirect suggestion succeeds at such points, it succeeds in terms of the transference distortions. It serves in effect to reinforce the defense against anxiety. In such circumstances the outcome can only rest on shifting sands, since it depends for its stability on the secure maintenance of the distortion. And this would be a rather peculiar result to be accorded the status of a psychoanalytic objective.

Three years after Freud had made his brief comments on the transference phenomenon in his study of Dora, Ferenczi published his outstanding paper, "Introjection and Transference," in which he emphasized that neurotic dependency was central to transference. "The neurotic," he wrote in that paper, "is constantly seeking for objects with whom he can identify himself, to whom he can transfer feelings, whom he can thus draw into his circle of interest, i.e. introject." [16] Consequently, an analytic approach which neglects positive transference on conscious principle from the very outset also neglects the unconscious side of dependency, suggestibility or introjection. When the effects are apparently favorable, they will actually leave the patient where he was before the therapeutic contact, except that his unconscious dependency will have been reinforced by its recurrence with the analyst.

If Freud were correct in his view that he rediscovered suggestion in the shape of transference, then it would follow that psychotic and schizophrenic processes in which relatedness and communication are so grossly distorted should be most amenable to suggestion; presumably, the greater the transference, the greater the accessibility to suggestion, for, as Thompson notes, the difference

[16] S. Ferenczi, *Sex in Psychoanalysis*, New York: 1950, pp. 47-48.

between neurotic and psychotic transference is that far more of
the psychotic's behavior is transferred distortions.[17] But it is palpably not the case that the psychotic is most amenable to suggestion. Because such patients are refractory to suggestion Freud
decided that analytic therapy would never be successful with
other than the transference neuroses in which the inner resistances could be overcome with the help of suggestion.[18] His
method of analyzing transference, then, was to create a therapeutic situation in which suggestion—originally the tool of hypnosis—could be effective; but he never specified whether the mode
of suggestibility was of any consequence.

The more entrenched and pervasive the distortion the less
amenable it is to suggestion of any sort; and it cannot simply
be overcome because it always contains an incontrovertible ingredient of truth in it. A therapeutic approach which requires
any sort of unconscious process to be overcome will eventually
serve as a corrective instrumentality. It will consolidate, enlarge
and strengthen the very thing it was designed to overcome.
Without conceiving of transference distortions in the wider context of accompanying feelings—doubts, fears and anxieties—the
analyst cannot approach it constructively and beneficially. When
faced with this clinical situation, Freud threw up his hands and
separated the transference neuroses from the narcissistic neuroses; his new technique would only work with patients whose
ready suggestibility was open and inviting during the transference experience. Why it was necessary to develop a new technique to achieve this end is not altogether clear, in view of the
fact that hypnotism could gain equally direct access to the repressed by the same means of suggestion. What is quite clear today, however, is that his use of suggestion during positive transference overlooked the wider context of the resistance that sets
it in operation. This may be confirmed by the fact that it is necessary to obtain a larger picture of the defensive operation where

17 C. Thompson, "Sullivan and Psychoanalysis," in P. Mullahy (ed.), *The
Contributions of Harry Stack Sullivan*, New York: 1952, p. 105.
18 Reference footnote 1, p. 394.

suggestion during positive transference does not fulfill the expectations of Freud's technique.

Having established, where suggestion is futile, that attendant
anxiety must be analyzed in conjunction with the resistance, we
know now that suggestion was also therapeutically useless even
where it yielded results which satisfied the patient, his close ones
and the therapist's conception of a well adjusted person. When
these underlying anxieties were not tapped and explored, such
suggestion during positive transference only added another coat
of whitewash to the unconscious dependencies and made them
even less accessible to awareness than they were before the apparently therapeutic suggestion was made. Overcoming resistances in order to gain access to the repressed traumata may have
secured the expression of repressed materials; but this was secured at the expense of repressing the resistances—the defensive
context of anxiety—by the effective use of suggestion. To put it
in another way, Freud's technique made for the suppression of
function to achieve the expression of content. The function of
resistance is to avoid anxiety, and when the resistance was itself
suppressed, it carried with it the therapist's avoidance of the patient's avoidance of anxiety. In this turn of psychological events,
the patient accomplished exactly what his resistance was supposed
to accomplish in interpersonal relations, only this time it was done
with the therapist's assistance. In psychological therapy as else-
where an authoritarian technique generates as its counterpart a
desire to elude authority and pursue what one requires of himself in secret if necessary, especially where the authority's mode of
operation, while not permitting free expression, is in complete
accord with it.

Freud had developed this technique of transference analysis
in a conceptual framework which was laden with unregenerate
vestiges of hypnosis. In this connection, however, Ferenczi was far
less equivocal in his view that "not only is analysis not any kind
of suggestion but a constant battle against suggestive influences,
and that the technique of analysis uses more protective measures
against blind belief and unquestioning submission than any

methods of teaching and enlightenment that have ever been used
in the nursery, the university or the consulting-room." [19] The
analysis of transference is thus the opposite of suggestion in hypnosis or anywhere else: it does not depend on the patient's parataxic
suggestibility to effect a cure. If the latter is all that can be done,
there is little more to be said about it. But, of course, "the pure
gold of analysis," [20] in one of Freud's favorite phrases, requires
that transferences, no matter their quality in the analyst's judgment, be studied to the point where the patient can do future
analyses of them himself and eventually not have to go through
with such transference involvements at all. This view is based on
the assumption that people who undergo analysis, despite vicissitudes in the transference relationship, really want to understand
themselves in order to lead happier lives. It is based on faith in
the human desire for self-knowledge and secure satisfactions.

[19] S. Ferenczi, *Further Contributions to the Theory and Technique of Psychoanalysis*, London: 1925, p. 66; also pp. 228–229. This was originally written in 1912, some six years before Freud published his view.

[20] S. Freud, "Turnings in the Ways of Psychoanalytic Therapy," *Collected
Papers*, Volume II, London: 1924, p. 402.

chapter six

Past and Future in the Present

CLASSICAL ANALYSIS SINCE FREUD has been more interested in problems of childhood—that is, of the pre-oedipal and oedipal phases—than in any other period of life. When he wrote, "If the physician should be specially connected . . . with the father-imago, it is quite in accordance with his actual relationship to the patient," [1] he took cognizance of the initial character of the therapist-patient relationship as an actual prototype of a parental "imago"; hence the problems of childhood which are evoked by experiences of authority. But he did not proceed to other periods of development and observe that "imagos" experienced throughout life may be projected onto the analyst. To be sure, any thorough investigation of any disturbance must consider early parent-child relationships, but this is not the whole story. And since we do not subscribe to the view that there is a core to neurosis which has a single magical resolution, the working through of any one distortion is as useful and beneficial as the working through of any other so far as the analytic process is concerned.

Realistically, of course, an analyst does represent the discipline of psychoanalytic science and art. He presumably knows more about some things than his patients and is presumably skilled in utilizing this knowledge. The therapeutic relationship is initially structured by him. Fees, place, time, frequency and so on are actually dependent upon the contingencies of the analyst's schedule, the location of his office or place of employment, his need for money, status or whatever. The patient has very little control of these things once he decides on a certain analyst. Moreover, the patient—it is hoped realistically—seeks help from the analyst; he wants something he feels he is supposed to get and this im-

[1] S. Freud, "The Dynamics of the Transference," *Collected Papers*, Volume II, London: 1924, p. 313–314.

mediately sets the stage for transference distortions of early childhood. In a setting such as this problems with parents or parental surrogates are most easily touched off. Unconscious habitual attitudes developed during the juvenile, pre-adolescent and adolescent periods of life are not as readily susceptible to being evoked by the initial structuring of the therapeutic situation.

The initial phases of transference usually comprise distortions from early development. The analyst's skill comes to the fore in this connection in order to widen the inquiry into difficulties of other developmental periods. It requires his divesting himself of socially defined accoutrements which confer authority upon him. It requires his willingness to enter the situation as one human being prepared to speak uncircuitously to another human being. This is a simple truism which is therapeutically useful just because it would be true even if it were not necessary for movement in the analytic process. It paves the way for an equalitarian relationship which the patient was capable of during pre-adolescence but may never have had the opportunity to experience; and he has to listen to it a number of times in different contexts before he will begin to hear it. To concentrate exclusively or predominantly on problems with parental authorities or oedipal factors as transference phenomena will hamper the patient's learning that he can, as a self-respecting person, authorize his own behavior without necessarily being obstructed by the enmity, hostility, envy or destructiveness of others.

The sharp focus on childhood distortions may be defended on the ground that they are the earliest and presumably the most binding in the growth of personality. But the clarification of distortions from whatever period in life is equally important. The actual difficulties one encounters currently living through a distortion are, moreover, of greater moment than simply delineating the historical context in which it may have been molded and established. For it is impossible to go back in time and relive the earlier situations with the knowledge one has gained from the present, and, consequently, the unlived future in which the distortions have yet to be made is the compelling locus of analytic therapy. Holding this future possibility open on a realistic basis is the most an analyst can do to concretize and enlarge a patient's hopes for improvement and change. There is a sense of finality about the past; the future is open and inviting to new modes of adaptation. The suffering one can yet avoid in life has more meaning and purpose for the analysis of psychological limitations than the suffering which is past and irretrievable.

Classical psychoanalytic method relied on free association. To be sure, a direct approach to the patient's current problems would have incurred his distortions very quickly and would thus have deprived the analyst of any leverage from the past to consider them as distortions. But the free-association-on-the-couch technique created special difficulties in the reconstruction of infantile neuroses. Aside from personal predilections, Freud originally defended the use of the couch as a means to avoid "all imperceptible influences on the patient's associations . . . so that the transference may be isolated and clearly outlined when it appears as resistance." [2] This view of his is difficult to understand because when he wrote it he had already realized that the analyst had to be analyzed. Personal analysis has proved to be of incalculable utility for enlarging the analyst's awareness of his effects on the developments of transference. Experience has shown, moreover, that this clear delineation of transference is not impeded when the patient sits up. In fact, perceptible and imperceptible influences on transference manifestations are not only unavoidable; these interactions of analyst and patient really provide opportunities for intense transference experiences out of which something worthwhile can emerge. I once thought it would be a crucial experiment to have the arrangements for treatment made by a receptionist and have the analyst sit behind a one-way vision screen. This would eliminate his influences and allow the distortions to develop in a pure state, whatever that would mean. But it obviously could not work because the analyst would occasionally have to say something to his patient and if he did not, the

[2] S. Freud, "Further Recommendations in the Technique of Psychoanalysis," *Collected Papers*, Volume II, London: 1924, p. 354.

transference distortions would develop in relation to the receptionist.

The shortcomings of the free-association-on-the-couch technique become clear indeed from Freud's study of the "Wolf-man," a patient whose pronounced passive dependency translated itself into a transference relationship which prolonged therapy indefinitely.[3] It should be mentioned that there were other factors—acknowledged scientific interest and loans of money—which also fostered the prolongation of treatment in this particular case. None the less, suspension of critical judgment had predisposed the analytic work to the emergence of fantasies and recollections of the past, some of which Freud once found were concocted for his benefit. The genetically oriented focus of the interpretations also favored this tendency. In fact, classical method placed at the disposal of patients two kinds of operations which militated against the analysis of transference: They could easily avoid the current difficulties in living which originally brought them to treatment, since the emphasis on genetic reconstruction played right into it. They were also enabled to act out many feelings, resurrected by genetic exploration, in their current experience without having to assimilate such feelings in their present character organization simply because the analyst was interested in delving into infantile conflicts; the "displaced affects" eluded investigation because they did not, with the analyst's express agreement, come under the purview of therapeutic interest.

The actual situations of the past in which the damaging experiences originated and developed are really gone and finished. Their enduring conditioning effects, however, are met again in the therapeutic situation, and they can be analyzed as probable effects on the course of future experience. It may be laid down that no distortion, as created under past conditions, can as such be satisfied in the context of the present, no matter how thoroughly it is analyzed. Certain unsatisfied demands of the past will always remain unsatisfied; those deprivations cannot be retrieved

[3] S. Freud, "From the History of an Infantile Neurosis," *Collected Papers* Volume III, London: 1925, pp. 473–605.

and fulfilled with current surrogates; that time has passed, those opportunities are gone. The particular circumstances which made them possible goals of action at that time will probably never occur again in one's life-history. They are revived in analysis to the end that they be seen as hopeless goals which will never be attained in their original state. To pursue those possibilities of satisfaction may provide one with a sense of goal-oriented behavior because they have not yet been tested and acknowledged to be unrealizable. But side by side with this persistent quest is the persistence of situations in which it bore no fruit—a reciprocal repetition of quest and failure. Losing hope in the realization of this impossible goal, the patient must feel hopeless and helpless, not necessarily as a child but as any repeatedly frustrated person who must now discover new ways of living in order to find hope again, and realizable possibilities for love. These feelings of hopelessness, usually accompanied by rage and hatred, are probably as significant as neurotic needs for love.

The idea of transforming repetition into recollection and into recollection alone implied that the present and future were to be studied in the perspective of the past, that the present and future were not viewed in their own right and that the past was not to be studied in their perspective.[4] But the alternative principle that human experience has forward movement as its direction makes it equally important to understand the past from the perspective of the future. Freud took account of it in his theoretical formulations about the topography of personality even though he never translated his divisions of id, ego and superego into principles of therapeutic practice. He finally began to recognize in theory that the meaning of the past did not exhaust all of the meaning of human life but he failed to reconstruct his therapeutic conceptions to make room for these later insights. One need not accept his threefold division of personality as the best heuristic model of personality organization to realize that he saw this. If these separate divisions are taken functionally and temporally, they refer

4 See, also, B. Wolstein, "Transference: Historical Roots and Current Concepts in Psychoanalytic Theory and Therapy, *Psychiatry*, XXIII (1960), pp. 159–171.

in a rough sense to what we now understand by impulse, intelligence and habit. For this heuristic model contains clues to the reconstruction of his theory of transference; it implies the liberation of transference conceptions from exclusive concern with the goals of hypnotherapy.

What one has done, what one wants done and what one expects to do are all interwoven into the fabric of any decision at any particular point in one's life history. The id in the dynamic sense of impulse, the ego in the sense of current workings of intelligence, and the superego in the sense of habitual organizations of impulse and intelligent direction all have a dual perspective in which they are to be viewed: how they have operated in the past and how they may operate in the future.[5] When the conscious-unconscious distinction is introduced, the situation becomes rather complicated because every significant occasion in which impulse, intelligence and habit converged was also a possible occasion for the experience of anxiety and attendant need to limit and assuage this unpleasant experience; and every such occasion contained the possibility of modifying the experience with what has been variously named as resistance, defense mechanism and security operation. By viewing the intensive study of personality in these terms, we are enabled to see that psychological processes which have become laden with anxiety in the past and have therefore become intolerable may also have a future reference despite the fact that the defensive operation was instituted in the past. Thus impulse, intelligent decision and organized habit were all capable of being arrested in their development and expression and all of them pointed to specific occasions in the past so far as Freud's therapeutic conception was concerned. But these arrested processes also have a future reference in what he expects to do in his life; and their future reference is of course immediately apparent when they are not arrested.

Now if we psychoanalysts are participant observers, it means that we cannot overlook this forward movement in the patient's

[5] See B. Wolstein, "Dewey's Theory of Human Nature," *Psychiatry,* XII (1949), pp. 77–85. Also, see *Appendix A* (1964), pp. 208–211, for implications of this view in the development of psychoanalytic procedure.

life; and if we follow the patient in our attempts to understand him, we must study his life-processes as he experiences them rather than concentrate on applying a specific conception of what is wrong with him.

Thus far, this inclusion of future expectations has been based on the fundamental limitations of Freud's hypnotic conception. But the importance of the future for the analytic process can easily be justified in its own terms. If we recognize the need to work through dynamic considerations during treatment, we also have to recognize the forward propulsion of any dynamism; it is going somewhere and the patient might be interested in finding out where it is going; and this is nothing more than an explicit interest in what the patient is trying to do in his life. It may make him anxious to consider the future course of his life, and this is all right if he learns what about it makes him anxious. Besides, it is this anxiety which brings him into analysis in the first place, and to fail to take cognizance of it would deny us an important basis for constructive analytic therapy. For the patient will never actually have to face and relive his failures and disappointments which occurred long ago and far away; an obsessive preoccupation with such events might even be investigated just because such failures and disappointments can never be recaptured and undone. Clarity about the past which lacks live connections with current doings and sufferings can only lead to a mechanical manipulation of the future anyway.

It may be stated categorically that any patient who has little anxiety about what will happen in the course of his life will be a poor treatment risk and that the initial possibilities of constructive collaboration are minimal. When a patient is exclusively concerned with what has troubled him in the past—and where this concern is not a response to his reading of Freud and other genetically oriented psychoanalysts—one must either say that he is feverishly defending himself against facing what his future holds or that his future is so dismal that he will be able to do very little about it even if he does develop a clear understanding of the factors responsible for how he got that way. In fact, it is highly doubtful that this understanding will develop in a clear state anyway.

Freud's idea that transference be utilized to persuade the patient to meet again and overcome the difficulties of the past thus requires careful modification. His view of the matter—to transform repetition into recollection—reflects a one-sided interest in the recollection of the past; it does not bridge the gap between past difficulties and present experiences; and it certainly ignores the future life-course of the patient. It's like walking backwards to go forward without looking where one's going, seeing only what has been left behind as the basis for going ahead. But just as the past spontaneously finds its way into the future, using transference as a bridge, so the future penetrates backward into the past and shapes the transference. Past difficulties are not mechanically repeated in a contemporary vacuum. The contemporary components of transference—experiences of the analyst and the day's events—cannot of course be separated from genetic development. On the other hand, the exclusive preoccupation with genetic determinants simply to transform repetition into recollection will divert the inquiry from current expectations and future purposes. Past and present go hand in hand, and the future extends itself from the present.

It is frequently observed that transference distortions are underway before the analyst is seen, just as the distortions have been operating before psychoanalysis was even considered. Thompson's early insistence that the transference relationship with the analyst is never completely distorted made the patient's contemporary perceptions as much a part of analytic therapy as his past perceptions of his parents.[6] What the patient has heard about analysis and the analyst he expects to consult and what took place during their first phone contact usually supply him with enough clues to start the transference process going. These initial contacts touch off distortions which were molded by cultural accidents of

[6] C. Thompson, "Development of Awareness of Transference in a Markedly Detached Personality," *International Journal of Psychoanalysis,* XIX (1938), pp. 299–309.

birth and biography. And the analyst cannot claim that they have nothing at all to do with him. As a professional person in an ostensibly laissez faire society, he has certain cultural characteristics which typify his group; and he has certain personal characteristics, as a particular member of this group, which cannot be blotted out of his communication and relatedness with others. Both of these types of factors, socio-cultural and personal, provide the patient with springboards for distortion, and he can use his knowledge for constructive as well as destructive ends. To deny the existence of these factors—the so-called reality factors in the therapeutic relationship from the analyst's side—is to deny entirely the validity of the patient's perceptions. Certain aspects of these perceptions are comparatively clear and veridical, and outright denial of this fact will do more harm than good for the later clarification of distortions.

Because it is often found that the original experiences were valid enough as experiences go, current distortions consist in the enduring quality of past conditioning experiences in decidedly unrelated situations. These past experiences lose their pastness, leave their moorings in the historical series of situations in which they took form, and tend to operate freely in the present by glossing over crucial traits of the current environment or perceiving them in special ways. These experiences with the analyst are focal points for both pushing back into history and pushing forward to purposes, goals and expectations. A prevailing transference process, then, requires an interpretive placement of its multiple aspects in the career-line from which it emerged; it also requires a constructive placement of its probable functions in the eventual life-course into which it proceeds. As Fromm-Reichmann states it, "Dissolution of parataxic misjudgments can best be done through the medium of investigating distortions in patients' interpersonal experiences with the psychiatrist." [7] This statement implies the interpenetration of past and future in the present,

[7] F. Fromm-Reichmann, *Principles of Intensive Psychotherapy*, Chicago: 1950, p. 98.

and Fromm-Reichmann certainly avoids the pitfalls of Freud's concept of transference neurosis in which a new set of neurotic distortions is created.

In the earlier days of analysis, when transference factors derived from infancy and childhood were given foremost consideration, historico-genetic analysis was designed to trace the problem back to its ultimate origins, using suggestion all the way to overcome resistance to recall. With the trauma of birth the biological dead-end of this approach was reached; the swing in technical interest could only move in one direction and that was forward. The past cannot be studied for its own sake, whatever that would mean; we study the past the better to manage the present in the light of future expectations. Since the genetic approach alone cannot study the persistence of any social or natural process, it cannot serve as the analytic method of studying psychological processes either. Since the modification of a process requires that its origins be reconsidered in terms of its expected course, the method of psychoanalysis must be genetic-functional. For historico-genetic analysis, with or without hypnotic suggestion, failed to encompass aspects of life as it is lived.

Past and future interpenetrate in the current unfolding of interpersonal processes, and this calls for an appropriate method for dealing with them, a genetic-functional one. The approach in psychoanalytic therapy is trifaceted or trifocal. It encompasses their genetic career and development through various life-situations, their current operation as a disturbance in relation to other people, and future conditions which obviate or include them in a satisfactory way. Which of these aspects is underscored depends on what is being studied at any particular point in analytic therapy. I want to emphasize that this genetic-functional or operational approach to the technique of psychoanalytic therapy does not lay down initially which phase is paramount; the definition of the problem really decides which line of inquiry is to be used in the concrete situation. The genetic phase is not tacked on out of homage to Freud; nor is the functional phase tacked on out of rejection of the genetic one. Both are equally important and cooperating phases of a single methodology—but not one to the exclusion of the other.

To study genesis apart from function would foster the minute recollection of the instigating factors without any attempt to rectify the current disturbances. To study current function apart from genesis would only resolve, and mechanically at that, some transient manifestations of a difficulty which may again appear unchanged in another unstudied situation. The more problematic and troublesome the process the greater the likelihood that the inquiry will concentrate not so much on present function and future purpose as on genetic circumstances and past developments. Both the analyst and the patient want to know how it got that way. They are interested in its general course of growth through the vicissitudes in the life-career of the patient to date. Once this is thoroughly scrutinized, there is a return to its present function, for the genetic interest was originally governed by a desire to envisage future situations in which the characteristic incidence of those disturbances will have been mitigated or averted.

The application of genetic-functional method is an art but the rationale of its methodology is clear. It is designed to avoid two widely different kinds of power-struggle which have been nurtured by two different approaches in analytic therapy. In Freud's predominantly genetic approach, the objective was to relate current difficulties to infantile sources and explain them on that basis. The current operation of those difficulties was left to itself, and tacit assent was given to their continuation. To cast a person's entire post-infantile experience into the mold of an infantile framework requires not only dialectical agility on the part of the analyst but a certain docility on the part of the patient. Without an affectionate transference the struggle that was bound to ensue could only be curtailed by recognition of the analyst's authority; the therapeutic relationship would otherwise be destroyed.

Freud's early training in hypnotism had probably remained with him in this decision to overcome the resistances instead of analyzing them. He was essentially interested in the content of repression on the cathartic assumption that reproduction of the repressed with appropriate affect would entail a basic change in the patient's personality structure. But this usually did not take place. It was observed time and again that the treatment worked but patients did not change for the better. Our proposal to unify genesis and function is not in accord with the genetic point of view which Freud held, for he was interested in overcoming resistances in order to get at the infantile content of the conflict. Of course, function and content cannot be divorced from each other in the processes of relatedness and communication. But a crucial change in focus has been made which places the remembered materials in a different perspective: For example, the fact that a certain type of fantasy follows upon an anxiety attack is as important as the content carried in the fantasy itself; getting involved in the content of the fantasy may actually interlock with the patient's half-conscious attempt to avoid anxiety, for he had engulfed it with a fantasy; the analyst can only communicate a desire to reinforce this avoidance if, by the dictates of his analytic technique, he finds the content of the fantasy more fascinating than the simple fact that it assuages and contains anxiety.

Our concern with genesis, consequently, is to connect genesis and function of the very resistances which Freud tried to remove in order to get at what he considered the problem. The aim of genetic-functional method is to study the genesis and function of these very resistances or defensive operations, while the content of the problem—infantile or current, real or imagined—is taken as a clue to the ways they organize anxiety.

The other kind of power-struggle develops out of the exclusively functional approach which is found in Horney's therapeutic method. She defined the main neurotic disturbances in terms of the consequences of neurotic trends; and her therapeutic objective was first to hit upon the neurotic trends and then to outline their detailed functions and consequences.[8] Such direct confrontation of the patient's characteristic disturbances can easily be

8 K. Horney, *New Ways in Psychoanalysis*, New York: 1939, pp. 280–282.

experienced by him as a challenge. "As I see it," she wrote, "the special challenge of the psychoanalytical situation consists in the fact that the patient's customary defensive attitudes cannot be used effectively. They are uncovered as such, thus forcing to the foreground the repressed trends underlying these defenses." [9] To challenge the patient is to evoke a mosaic of defenses. This may be useful as a time-saving device and may bring to light many of the repressed trends which might otherwise remain repressed for a much longer period. But it does not contribute much more to the successful analysis of defenses and the repressed trends underlying them. It does not provide a base for their understanding and control in the feeling knowledge of the patient, it will probably fail because therapeutic results on purely functional bases are integrated in a mechanical way, perhaps even in the manner of a post-hypnotic suggestion.

Horney's direct approach to the patient was a challenge which can be construed as an accusatory, guilt-producing device. This is inferred from her failure to inquire why the direct challenge was itself necessary in order to call the patient's attention to the consequences of his behavior. In fact, she went back to Freud's first technique of psychotherapy which he had used with Emmy von N. But she did it without the use of the hypnotic trance as an adjunct to her method.

In a dominantly functional procedure the analyst assumes that he has much more cognitive power than he actually possesses; and when he must do it, he will. But the patient is burdened with responsibilities which he cannot really be held accountable for. He does not have the required understanding to assume these responsibilities, since he has been enjoined by the method from knowing which origins are significant for which consequences; and he finds himself having to accept an authoritative judgment about something he is in no position to understand. If the patient does, on this approach, change his patterns of behavior, these changes are generally mechanical. For they have very little

9 Reference footnote 8, pp. 163–164.

groundwork laid in his own understanding of life. He can only
continue on this suggested basis and hope that no unexpected occurrence will require that he think over his life-course for himself in quest of further understanding.

Thus Horney's "hypnotism" was to analyze the defenses without providing the patient with an opportunity to develop a
backdrop in his own experience against which to feel and understand their operation. The patient knew why he did what he did
but he had acquired this knowledge on the analyst's say-so. He
did what he had to do, knew why he did what he had to do but
he could not reorganize his activities unmechanically because
his span of understanding had been circumscribed by the analytic
approach, and he had been denied levers from the past to consolidate his own feelings and thoughts for self-realization.

It may be the unfortunate lot of all innovators to become so
enamored of their departures from earlier investigators that they
throw the baby out with the bath in order to start afresh. This
technical discovery that psychological disturbances have current
functions and characteristic consequences as well as historical
sources in repression may have made it necessary for Horney to
differentiate her contribution very sharply from the exclusive
concern with genesis. It must of course be remembered that this
technical advance is of definite aid in clarifying the currently
disturbing factors when it does not introduce a prevailing atmosphere of challenge and power-struggle into the analytic situation;
nor can it be overlooked that this development also stemmed
from the rejection of Freud's biologized, mechanical and deterministic psychology. But in analytic technique, there is no possible choice of either exclusive concern with the genesis of psychological difficulties or exclusive concern with their functions
and consequences.

The denial of genetic considerations which Horney brought
into vogue was probably intended as a means to counterbalance
Freud's sole genetic aim of recovering lost memories. But it contained a certain confusion: To deny that the recall of past content is in itself the effective factor in analytic therapy is one

thing; but to deny on principle that the patterns in which that content has been integrated can have effects on later life is quite another thing; and the latter—Horney's view—would imply that the functions and consequences of those past effects are to be eliminated from the analyst's sphere of interest.

A genetic-functional approach is essential for a thoroughgoing analysis of complex and intimate connections between past effects and anticipated consequences. When either the genetic or functional is taken exclusively, it produces a one-sided approach. Freud looked largely to past content for crucial data and Horney considered nothing but actual function and consequences as the crucial data. The kind of data Horney considered significant—neurotic trends, as she called them—is still considered more significant than the mere recall of traumatic events. But the psychoanalytic approach to their clarification is different; there is instead a continual working back and forth between their genesis and function.

In these two sorts of power-struggle which can occur, the analyst may, if his approach is adaptive to the communicational currents, find a way to turn the trend of investigation to constructive therapeutic ends. Not so much by a syntaxic confrontation of the patient's defensive operations but rather by an inquiring attitude about the exclusive use of past or present. This inquiry into what prompts or stimulates the specific line of communication often elicits very interesting information, some of which might prove to be rather instructive to those who take a one-sided approach. For example, the patient who continually discusses events in the past may sometimes frankly report that he does it in order not to have to face his feelings about his daily experiences with various people, including the analyst. This use of past reports acts as a kind of support for his customary system of attitudes and beliefs that originally instigated him to seek out analytic help. If the analyst remains a sympathetic listener in such circumstances, he actually reinforces the patient's troubled system of operations, reaffirming their validity rather than opening up the troubled spots. Another sort of patient may be constantly

preoccupied with present experiences and current feelings toward the analyst. He can spend session after session discussing
current life-experiences and even point out the anxieties which
accrue to them in a very objective manner. Occasionally, he will
even resent the analyst's search for historical information to put
these difficulties into intelligent focus and make the anxieties
meaningful and experienceable in the present; for the objective
description of feelings serves as a defense against investigating
current experiences of feeling.

In brief, Freud tried to overcome resistances and lay bare the
infantile conflicts. On the other hand, Horney rejected the study
of infantile conflicts, and tried to study the consequences of those
resistances without studying their origins. The genetic-functional
approach, as defined here, goes along with Horney in rejecting
the exclusive focus on the content of infantile conflicts. It goes
along with her in making transference distortions the subject matter of analytic therapy. However, it sustains the significance of
past resistances in the study of their functional consequences. At
the current stage of our knowledge, the operation of neurotic
trends cannot be defined merely in terms of functions and consequences; its definition requires the interpenetration of genesis
and function.

I propose the use of this term "genetic-functional" to describe
this method of analytic therapy. It is extremely well-suited for
this purpose because it encompasses the important temporal
phases of all interpersonal processes with which psychoanalysts
deal. It entails at once the past and the future in present aspects
of processes, and it points up their temporal, continuous, cumulative and purposive character.

Interpersonal processes have histories; they have beginnings,
middles and ends. Like historical occurrences, they are ultimately
unique, individual, induplicable and singular. They cannot be
understood apart from the circumstances to which they accrue
and in which they operate. Fortunately, we only have to deal with
interpersonal processes in the short run. We do not have to acquire any ultimate and absolute understanding of them, for in

the long run we die and our problem-solvings are over; it is none the less true that our deaths may become issues of moment for close ones as well as ourselves, and so these events in their natural or unnatural course may in turn become matters demanding attention. However, since no two life-situations are exactly alike as constituted and construed in all of their particulars, each psychological process acquires its own specific traits. Each feeling and attitude must be understood in its own particular constellation of feelings and attitudes as well as in its own concrete set of socio-cultural relations, two sides of the same coin as it were.

But interpersonal processes may be compared with historical events in another and more significant way: Their effects and meanings may continue to operate even after the situation in which they occurred has terminated. Their occurrence may be quite unique and induplicable, but their acquired meanings and influences persist in later life and change with exigent changes in outlook and purpose. As events that occurred at one time, they are ultimate facts; as ongoing processes, they may take on new characters and significances. They are passing occurrences which can wittingly or unwittingly be retained in memory and be effective in behavior. Their meanings can change when current foci in conscious awareness change.

The only pasts and futures of which we are aware are those which arise in the current foreground of experience.[10] This statement may sound like a truism but it throws into sharp relief the fact that everyone continually rewrites his personal history at crucial points in his life-course. This history is the only history he has of himself but it can always be rewritten. The fact of this potentiality is not always discernible. It is perhaps most clearly discerned in a problematic situation where the understanding of both past experience and future expectation is ensnarled by current disruptions, distortions and disturbances.

10 The fact of continuity, therefore, is a condition for survival, and not a cause nor an explanation. For further comments on this view that knowledge of the present opens up the understanding of the past, see S. Hook, "A Pragmatic Critique of the Historico-Genetic Method," in *Essays in Honor of John Dewey*, New York: 1929.

chapter seven

A Formulation of the Concept

THAT THE ANALYST has an active role in therapeutics is no secret, and Freud was well aware of it. If the clear statement of these very involved issues was his difficulty, then it is true that he had done enough to have blazed the trail. However, the worth of his therapeutic conceptions must be tested against current theory and experience, and he would have been the first to demand rigorous examination of his early views. Today, we may believe that he did not exactly say what he meant; but we must, in all fairness, take him to have meant only what he said. And it is this meaning which is being explored.

There is a somewhat neglected aspect to the development of psychoanalytic technique which is rather curious and even somewhat ironic. The analyst was of course construed as a mirror reflecting to the patient only what the patient had said; he was construed as a depersonalized observer. But some technical formulations were couched in terms which convey much more than that, especially those concerning positive and negative transference and resistance. The patient transferred oedipal feelings to the analyst which the analyst then judged as positive or negative. The patient resisted the analyst which indicated that the analyst's participation in the therapeutic situation was much more than that of a mirror. Most striking in this connection is the type and extent of activity which Freud enjoined upon the analyst—"guiding suggestion," "overcoming resistances" and so on—when, at the same time, he considered the analyst a passive mirror reflecting back to the patient only what he had heard.

As experience grew and theory was enlarged, the protection afforded the analyst by this classical construction was dropped and he was freed to enter very much into the interpersonal situation. An interesting twist to Freud's mirror concept of the analyst has been observed with increased frequency. Patients who are rather sophisticated about the literature and theories of psychoanalysis refer to this idea quite directly or by implication in order to maintain psychological distance from the analyst. The analyst is perceived as a professional worker like a surgeon or a dentist who is supposed to resolve problems without infringing upon any of the defensive operations to which the patient has become accustomed. Where the need to keep the analyst at a distance is keenly felt, these perceptions are not always quite so deliberate or kind. In verbalizing this mirror conception of the analyst, the patient is often communicating a mild form of dissociation of his distortions from his self-system, and so he dumps them in the analyst's lap and expects them to be resolved without any further involvement on his part.

The willingness of contemporary psychoanalysis to acknowledge the participation of the analyst in the inquiry has put a different complexion on these processes. The transference distortions are experienced in an interpersonal situation in which one person, the participant observer, ostensibly places his skills at the disposal of another, the observed participant, and these distortions convert it into an interpersonal situation in which the observer is not entirely the other person. The distortions are neither positive nor negative but simply irrational or parataxic, and the patient, rather than resisting the analyst, is actually impeding the emergence of his own insight in some complex fashion. This revised perspective threw into sharp relief the extent to which the patient was actually obstructed by his own distortions. It is now clearly seen that the analyst's personality provides points of attachment for both clear and distorted beliefs, and whether aspects of his personality are clear or distorted for him will determine the extent to which he will be able to respond to them in a therapeutically useful way.[1]

[1] C. Thompson, "Transference and Character Analysis," *Samiksa*, VII (1953), pp. 260–270. The implicit assumption is that the therapeutic undertaking can only go as far as an analyst is able to perceive distorted components in the patient's transference relations and communications.

When Freud abandoned hypnosis only to rediscover suggestion again in the form of transference, two important points were not entirely clarified: Transference in everyday life and analytic therapy can either involve an openness to syntaxic suggestion or import a distortion into perception; and transference distortions in analytic therapy, whether positive or negative, actually introduce blinders to syntaxic understanding and suggestion. The meaning of positive transference was never made clear in its intent. So far as Freud's usage was concerned, there is no reason to assume he did not mean unconscious material which we now consider worthy of therapeutic inquiry, though in his technique, so long as the distortion was positive and affectionate, it was not questioned on principle until it became resistance. In fact, on occasion, he did mean what we now consider to be a transference distortion. A good example of this is his discovery—or creation—of the transference-love phenomenon where all of the features of positive transference were left alone until one day they suddenly disappeared, and the analyst found himself in "a painful and embarrassing position." [2] But if we combine with these observations of transference-love his explicit injunction to skirt the theme of transference until after it had developed into resistance, this phenomenon becomes almost transparent. It was actually fostered by this curious blindness to its distorted quality just because it was deemed positive. In short, transference as distortion was not sharply distinguished from transference as an openness to syntaxic suggestion.

Transference is a complex mode of interpersonal relatedness and communication which goes on in life as well as in psychoanalytic therapy. It loses conceptual utility when applied to everyday life, since it is not ordinarily comprehended and since comprehension does not ordinarily lead to changes in personality. We analysts may well appropriate this term to denote specific manifestations of distorted and non-distorted attitudes, and for the sake of scientific clarity, restrict its usage to the communica-

[2] S. Freud, "Observations on Transference-Love," *Collected Papers*, Volume II, London: 1924, p. 381.

tional field in analytic therapy. It may be taken to refer to all such feelings and attitudes expressed toward the analyst. Syntaxic attitudes and parataxic distortions may be taken as the more general concepts which apply to life-situations as well as therapeutic ones, while transference is here used to refer solely to their operation in the therapeutic situation. This use of terms is perhaps arbitrary, but the distinctions involved are necessary. If one has other linguistic preferences for making these distinctions, there would be nothing to quibble about so long as these various matters retained their distinctive status.

A transference distortion is a vivid and telling experience. In this respect, it is similar to any other phase of relatedness and communication which may not be distorted. The experiences of transference distortion in therapy are as alive and as moving as any other kinds of experience which impell a person to action. If this were not so, there would be no accounting for the utility of transference analysis in the improvement of living. No transference experience is, on the other hand, entirely distorted, for at some points in the convergence of experience of two people, there must be factors or patterns of communication which make relatedness possible. This is much clearer with neurotic than with psychotic processes. Even prima facie, however, successful recapitulation of the career-line of psychotic and schizoid personalities would at least indicate that memory traces linger which make relatedness possible. Even if this were not logically demonstrable, it would have to be maintained as factually possible in a theory which is based on the possibility of therapeutic success with psychotics. It has to be maintained in theory because if the converse were true, namely that neurotic or psychotic transference phenomena are entirely distorted, there would be no basis in fact for communication. Any transference which has been analyzed with some success cannot have happened without some communicational toehold at some level of experience.[3]

[3] The concept of transference distortion embraces both neurotic and psychotic phenonema. Differences in technical approach to these diverse phenomena are dictated by a significant difference in the presenting features

Transference distortions are immediate, direct, unreflective and automatic reactions. They are habitual attitudes and feelings which are experienced under conditions of limited awareness. They reflect sharp limitations of psychological function imposed by anxiety. They limit the possibilities of seeing oneself and others as individuals in their own right, since newly encountered people become participants in the perpetuation of these indiscriminate reactions. They are largely refractory to the self-corrective antidote of intelligence and contemporary perception. They are retained in unknown fears and crystallized attitudes, the original motives and expected purposes of which are now beyond the reach of open and critical scrutiny.

I have distinguished between motive and attitude, and would like to digress and examine this distinction a bit further. An attitude is a crystallized organization of feelings and motives. Though many diverse feelings and conflicting motives are often combined in a distorted attitude, the analysis of conflict makes the unhampered expression of these feelings and motives possible. Psychoanalysis is chiefly concerned with such baggage from the past—habitual interpersonal attitudes which have lost their validity but still continue to function without the mediation of critical perception. This does not mean that the total personality disappears from the analytic situation and that these defensive attitudes are considered to the exclusion of feelings, fantasies and motives. The analyst is faced with a delicate decision when a break-through occurs, for often the patient, in his enthusiasm, will turn to an opposite extreme in defense against insight; this opposite extreme is not ordinarily seen to be itself determined by the unconscious process. None the less, in the analysis of habitual defensive attitudes, that is, compulsions, doubts, intellectualizations, hostility, simulated humor or transference-love, new potentialities for more contemporary experience begin to seep

---

which confront the therapist. In neurosis, the contracted evidence of distortion becomes magnified during the analysis of transference on the way to its resolution, while the gross evidences of distortion in psychosis are analyzed with the goal of contraction.

through. These potentialities are to be welcomed cordially rather than analyzed or judged because such reactivated motivations are the patient's own domain of experience. They are not discouraged or looked down upon; for these motives contain the seeds of new habitual attitudes which, being open to public inspection, may become malleable and flexible and under the control of the patient.

This distinction between feeling or motive on the one hand and habitual attitude or character armor on the other provides a conceptual basis for understanding how defensive operations become established. It helps to explain how certain habitual attitudes are broken through, how others may be established and how they become aligned with the compenetrating needs for spontaneity and stability. It also indicates how psychoanalysis is concerned with the future, for the goal of a motive becomes as important as its origin. A motive is literally what moves a person in his direction in life. As a concept, it embraces terms like feeling, fantasy or imaginative resources. The motive as named and conceptualized does not do the moving, however; the process to which we assign the status of "motive" does. The enlargement of awareness which comes from the genetic-functional analysis of motives would be self-defeating if it did not point to future possibilities of greater freedom and spontaneity in living. The liberation of imagination, motives and movements from the encumbrances of past experience and the expansion of their possibilities in new directions is, then, the desirable outcome of analyzing defensive attitudes.

When feelings and attitudes are introduced into a relationship in which they have no immediate other-personal counterpart, we can ascribe an initial inappropriateness to them. This does not mean that the meaningful content of all such feelings and attitudes is necessarily or ultimately inappropriate; but we must look into them, for even if they are eventually validated, we must ask why they were initially conveyed in this way. The unconscious aspects of the process are not restricted to the distorted personification of the analyst; a basic distortion of the patient himself and his perceptive capacities is also signified. The expression of a distorted personification of the analyst is instigated by interpersonal dynamics—that is, by past interpersonal situations which are consciously remembered or unconsciously lived through. Their referents are definitely not currently interpersonal in terms of the ongoing analytic situation, except perhaps in something the analyst is or says or does that touches off the remembrance of things past.

In the face of the unexperienced and unknown, the patient suffers severe limitations of objective reference which are aroused by anxiety; his habitual attitudes are disorganized. This is why his communications are with a personification sustained in those attitudes rather than with the person of the analyst. Since the other participant is not exactly the person sitting in the analyst's chair, the interpersonal situation has moved to a dynamic interpersonal status. And in this dynamic interpersonal situation the characteristic traits of the other person instigating and receiving a particular communication are not really present. It is in this sense that the distorted attitude is expressed in the personification of the analyst.

The patient's tendency to personify the analyst is located in his distorted perception of certain determinate personal attributes of the analyst. He usually has some inkling of its unconscious and uncomfortable qualities: His recognition that his communications have limited objective reference in the analytic situation, his recognition that he is really communicating with someone other than the personification sustained in and by his unconscious defensive attitudes, his eventual recognition of the validity of his objective perceptions of the analyst—all of these indicate that therapeutic transference is the development of an interpersonal situation in which some traits of the other person, the analyst, have become personified. The specific personality traits of the analyst become pegs, so to speak, on which these interpersonal experiences are hung, but as long as the analyst knows and can when necessary acknowledge relevant observations about his personal qualities, these distortions will, per se, have very limited reference to his actual personality organization. For if those feelings and attitudes are not actually evoked by the analyst, if their description is not manufactured by him—that is, if the patient's distortions are his own typical reactions but factually not in reaction to the analyst's activities, they will, to a large extent, be produced with any analyst. They will emerge in different forms depending on who the analyst is, but emerge they will—so long as the analyst's efforts at non-reciprocation do not interfere with his therapeutic interest, and so long as he does not fulfill the expectations of the personification, become parataxically realized and actually get enmeshed in the distortions.

There are no absolute and certain clinical criteria of distortion. From the standpoint of context, aims and development, the experiences of no two people are exactly alike. Because of this fact, the content of a process and its symbolic value are not in themselves reliable indices of its function. Two behaviorally similar events may have radically dissimilar motivational sources; what a man's behavior may mean to others is not always and may hardly ever be what it means to himself. General contructs have to be ventured about the regularities, patterns or organizations of that experience, however; and in virtue of this fact, a general formulation about the operation of transference distortions in analytic therapy can be constructed.

Transference distortions are usually touched off when the analyst attempts to probe materials which are beyond the patient's immediate awareness. When he undertakes an investigation of specific feelings or motives of past experience which are currently operating in a mesh of defenses, he loses his role as a skilled observer. He becomes the intersecting point of various personifications in the experience of a patient who has already become anxiously and defensively involved. If these personifications are carefully pursued with the patient, they will eventually be recognized to be the distortions they are. If, upon further inquiry, they are not revealed as distortions, and the analyst has sufficient self-awareness and security to acknowledge and confirm perceptions of himself which he identifies as being of himself, then it is the personality of the analyst rather than a personification which is experienced, and psychoanalysis is not ordinarily indicated. Very frequently, these accurate perceptions of the analyst also have a distorted side. These perceived qualities may be familiar to the patient, and he may find that they call forth specific sorts of automatic reactions which the analyst can safely say he does not require of anyone including the patient. And here analysis is indicated to study what automatically follows in response to it.

When these unconscious personifications can be traced to the patient's past, it used to be thought that a historical interpretation made at an emotionally urgent point would clarify them. It was called a mutative interpretation because it was supposed to modify the emotional situation when the patient heard that his transference distortions of the analyst repeated an oedipal pattern.[4] But unconscious processes are not ordinarily that compliant and such interpretations may actually confuse and block the further development of the emotional process being communicated. The patient may sometimes express an open reluctance to surrender modes of adaptation for which he has no ready substitutes even after he understands the logical connection of past and present, for they have been consolidated by their earned increments in the series of experiences with others prior to and concomitant with analytic therapy. The analyst's introduction of historical information cannot ordinarily resolve them. They must be continually lived through, repeatedly tested, alternately clutched and surrendered until their patent uselessness is demonstrated beyond a shadow of a doubt, and awareness of the problem, even then, can be reliable only after that awareness has withstood the test of time. Some patients have described this process as making the rounds of their problems, testing their fears, making the rounds again, testing again and so on with increasing clarification each time around. And this is essentially the point that Sullivan made in an unpublished lecture: " 'If the doctor doesn't get in the way, the context is run through the mill, and each time it

4 J. Strachey, "The Nature of the Therapeutic Action of Psychoanalysis," *International Journal of Psychoanalysis*, XV (1934) , pp. 127–159.

becomes a little clearer. That's the way obsessional personalities seem to heal themselves. They run their security operations over and over and over.' " [5]

No transference distortion, not even those of hysterical personalities, expends itself the way certain post-hypnotic suggestions do. It is designed to cope with undesirable features of experience and it matters little that current experiences may be grossly distorted. Occasionally, it runs its customary course again and again even when the patient has reliable knowledge that it is not called for by anything valid in the other person. By nature, all men desire to know, for knowledge liberates potentialities and yields power to act. And every transference distortion has its source and rationale in this search for mastery which is common to all men, the disturbing factor being that it persists beyond the consensually validated boundaries of contemporary experience.

The reason for the emergence of this state of affairs is easier to obtain than its resolution. Although the use of a defense may become largely conscious, its origin and purpose remain largely beyond current awareness. During transference, a patient usually recognizes that he is defensively involved. He usually has an idea of what he expects from the analyst—to impose goals, act destructively, be despotic or rejecting, demand certain acts in return for love and a host of other things, so he proceeds to protect himself against these eventualities in analysis with the knowledge that his defense will work again as it worked before. While the defensive operation may, thus far, be said to resemble post-hypnotic suggestion, the analogy breaks down at this point. A typical defensive operation has become firmly established over a long period of years in a variety of dissimilar situations. Though it may have caused much discomfort and restricted the possibilities of new experience, it also prevented the recurrence of the destructive integration with others, however distortedly perceived. Every neurotic trait, having been forged out of difficult experiences, has this dual aspect: it has aided the patient in maintaining a semblance

[5] M. J. White, "Sullivan and Treatment," *The Contributions of Harry Stack Sullivan*, New York: 1952, p. 135; by special permission of the W. A. White Psychiatric Foundation, Washington, D.C.

of integrity, on the invalid—or at least untried—assumption that everybody will want to repeat the intolerable experiences with him, and it has become an enduring trait in his personality structure.

Emotional intelligence is not easily achieved, perhaps because the basic structures of emotional life are not so obviously firm as the commonsense experience of the physical world. The life of feeling and emotion is, by sharp contrast, fluent and changing. There is a tendency to seek equilibrium to counter this flux. An established pattern, though it be distorted, is clung to rather tenaciously in order to avoid the risks of precariousness, novelty and the unknown. As a consequence, any "reality" which an individual has grasped and lived as true in the course of infinitely varied experience will become quite inured to any new "realities" which run counter to the enstated one.

If we hope that our patients will eventually learn new "realities" and respect their integrity, if we hope that they will respect their analytic experiences and allow them to crystallize, then they may rightfully expect us to respect the difficult experiences into which their distortions landed them prior to analysis. Respect for difficulties does not mean respect for distortions, however. Anyone who willingly subjects his life-experience to intensive scrutiny in cooperation with a psychoanalyst has arrived at a point in his life where he himself can no longer respect his distortions. For the analyst to respect a distortion would be about the same order of cooperation as a surgeon allowing an inflamed appendix to burst.[6] To state the analogy in other terms: We may

[6] The major deficiency of the non-directive approach is the therapist's insistence that he cannot, on principle, help the patient; this implies a respect for the distortion of the patient. But when this principle is made explicit in performance, non-directive therapy, contrary to its professions, also tries to help the patient. The non-directive group professes that it "defines the interview situation in terms of client responsibility for directing the interview"; yet in performance, the therapist is reported to make comments such as "Now suppose we consider that next time we get together and try to see what ways there are of developing that road" (C. Rogers, *Counseling and Psychotherapy*, New York: 1942, p. 121, 401).

quibble philosophically about the chicken-egg twister, but we know that given the egg the chick will follow. We cannot find fault with the chick just because it came from the egg, though we can, if we dislike chicks, interfere with the conditions under which eggs become fertile and hatch. Analysis may have sympathy for the results of distortions—that tragic magnitude of human waste; it may respect the potentialities people might have realized and, perhaps more important, what people may yet become; but it has no hospitality for distortions of perception.

Is the transference phenomenon a hypnotic one? Does it have any hypnotic elements or features about it? In view of the variety of observable distortions, it is important to dispose of whatever semantic difficulties are involved and get at the core of this matter. We can easily become embroiled in dialectics over the meaning and application of terms, whether the unconscious was a newer edition of the older hypnoid states and so on, but it is doubtful that semantic discussions prove much more than was originally assumed to be necessary and true. The repeatedly observable fact is that some transference distortions do appear to resemble post-hypnotic suggestions and that others have no traits in common with hypnotic phenomena; the former are the parataxic distortions in exactly the sense that Sullivan intended while the latter may be called derivative distortions. These derivative distortions are also parataxic in the sense that they obscure immediate perception of the environing conditions but they are simply derivations of defensive operations which would not have to be employed were it not for the fact that the defenses themselves were necessary in order to avert anxiety; they serve as precautions against the need to get the defenses into operation.

It is true that certain transference phenomena literally invite the hypnotic technique of suggesting away problems *in statu nascendi,* as Freud put it. These are the transference distortions from early childhood which developed in response to specific personality organizations and disorders of parents or parental surrogates. But they do not constitute the core of personality; they are the genetics of a process but not its functional results.

The analyst who has surrendered the hypnotic goals does not have to acknowledge the invitation to become another parental figure. His chief strength is his ability to differentiate himself at every crucial point from the personality of the real parent. In this way he avoids the pitfalls of the unsuccessful analysis of Dora where Freud failed to distinguish himself very sharply from Dora's father, and he places himself in the syntaxic position of being able to offer suggestions which stand on their own merits.

Despite qualitative and historical differences between derivative or precautionary defenses and the earlier ones, the analyst who will not play the hypnotic role may work exactly the same way in the face of both. His approach to any detected distortion can be uniformly analytic instead of being supportive and exhortative as if he were a parent, a guide, a pedagogue or anything of an authoritarian nature. Even the authority of psychoanalytic science is no final shibboleth simply because every patient has a kind of psychological laboratory in which to study interpersonal processes; and it might be recalled that every patient is potentially another Anna O. who may be able to teach psychoanalysis more about psychology than we already know. If the analyst harbors any strong supportive tendencies, he might keep them in check until he is reasonably sure that what he would like to support is relatively free of distortion.

It will be recalled that after Freud switched from cathartic method to the technique of free association, he continued to use suggestion against the resistances and seek the original content of early traumatic sexual experiences. His goals were still those of hypnosis; the authoritarian attitude of the analyst during positive transference was certainly the attitude of the suggestive hypnotist during the trance; and the underlying belief in the strict determination of mental events certainly played a significant part in both types of treatment. When transference manifestations appeared in this kind of psychoanalytic atmosphere, it was essentially correct, in view of these facts, to refer to hypnotic elements in transference.[7] Indeed, without such a charac-

[7] H. Nunberg, "Transference and Reality," *International Journal of Psychoanalysis*, XXXII (1951), pp. 1–9.

terization of Freud's thinking and working with transference, it would be impossible to make the therapeutic technique which he espoused intelligible.

Whether this condition was due to the limitations of technique or the restrictive influences of theory is difficult to make out from our present perspective. But wallowing in childhood fantasies to the exclusion of anything else was very clearly rationalized by the early pioneers in analytic therapy. Their point of view was supported by what they found in the anticipated transference distortions. They proceeded theoretically as if it were true that all unconscious processes in personality organization stemmed from early childhood. In virtue of their therapeutic procedure they were only able to observe and verify what they had originally expected to find in the evolving therapeutic process. They were able to conclude that the patient, in his analytic transference, was following out a parental command which was repressed long ago, while in post-hypnotic suggestion the subject was carrying out a command concerning which amnesia had been induced.[8]

These hypnotic elements appeared essentially because the analyst treated the patient in a child-like manner. The analytic procedure consisted in not being in any way a real person for the patient. The analyst tried as much as humanly possible to keep himself out of the situation, on the assumption that he could actually mirror the patient's communications without injecting anything of himself. In effect, he created a personification of himself to which the patient responded. The unreality of this personification and procedure eventually got communicated to the patient with the desired result that he developed a fantastic relationship with the analyst, these fantastic qualities being definitely rooted in the early maturation and acculturation of the child.

But there are other factors which have made an alteration in perspective necessary. We know that transference manifestations are not produced solely in virtue of the analytic procedure and

[8] S. Ferenczi, *Sex and Psychoanalysis*, New York: 1950, p. 76.

that they cannot be overcome by analytic injunction. They just happen as part of everyday interpersonal relationships; and transference distortions occur under analytic conditions essentially in virtue of the fact that the analyst is another human being. The conditions under which they occur—and the analyst's operant personality is definitely a part of those conditions—contribute to the character they acquire. And this is the kernel of truth that we can learn from clinical experience with the mirror method: what the analyst says and does is as important in the formation of transference distortions as the potential for typical sorts of distortion which the patient brings to analysis.

The analyst does not have to institute a "battlefield" on which to struggle with the patient's resistances; he may seek a situation in which the patient can learn the ins-and-outs of his anxieties and the distortions which obscure them. Though we do not deny the significance of uncovering the repressed in contemporary analysis, we no longer consider it as important as analyzing and acquiring a firm understanding of defensive or security operations. This consideration is based on the repeated observation that cathartic recall of repressed memories may afford the patient temporary emotional relief but it does not usually provide a solid basis for durable resolutions of disturbance in personality organization.

The therapeutic use of the patient's parataxic suggestibility during the so-called positive transference to transform repetition into recollection has highly questionable validity because the analyst-patient relationship can no longer be hypnotically conceived. As Rioch has shown, some transference reactions are similar to post-hypnotic suggestion.[9] The post-hypnotic effects of parental commands and demands made the early development of defensive patterns necessary for the integration of those injunctions with the child's emergent sense of self-esteem. Transference analysis has to study the enduring effects of such integrations, to demonstrate how the patient carries these integrations over into

[9] J. Rioch, "The Transference Phenomenon in Psychoanalytic Therapy," *Psychiatry*, VI (1943), pp. 147–156.

other situations with the expectation that others will make the same demands of him. The implicit presupposition of this procedure is that he can now participate in setting the conditions of his co-existence with others. Though he could not resist parental commands in early childhood, he no longer has to enact them or counteract them indirectly. The more he is free of the need to counteract past unwarranted intrusions by parents and others—counteractions which constitute transference phenomena in analysis—the less he will anticipate them in the present, the less he will have to obviate them in the future. Hence the post-hypnotic quality of distortions from early childhood. But the goals of analysis are no longer simply those of hypnosis because it is now evident that some transference distortions are not at all identical with any kind of hypnotic phenomena. To pursue the latter exclusively under psychoanalytic conditions would only call forth childhood attitudes and omit personality developments of the juvenile, pre-adolescent and adolescent eras where defensive operations which incur distortions do not have any observable hypnotic or post-hypnotic quality.

Transference phenomena emerge in a variety of ways throughout life to avoid intolerable episodes. Our therapeutic attempts to analyze them evoke a mosaic of defenses which preclude or limit openness and vulnerability to those hurts to which there has been no resistance; no resistance has generally proved intolerable; resistance even in the face of a friend who is interested in helping is more or less tolerable. And the problem is to demonstrate that resistance to certain expected reactions actually has little basis in the interpersonal experience with the analyst and that their chief basis for persistance rests in these expectations about his reactions. This very belief about expectations becomes an important factor in ordinary life-situations, though not—let us hope—in analysis. It can become a self-realizing proposition by seeking out the conditions which will make it come true and even producing the conditions where they do not exist to prove their truth.

Now if one has to call the occurrence of transferences in analysis hypnoid states or hypnoid elements, there is little more to be said about it. However, recent experience demonstrates quite clearly that this oversimplifies the nature of personality and its capacities for distortion. In so doing, it also conveys a distorted picture of the therapeutic task. It is not obligatory for the analyst to assume any particular attitude or personal quality when he works with patients; all he has to do is be himself and the transference distortions will occur. To create a specific type of therapeutic atmosphere by design tends to produce the conditions of hypnosis. The analytic situation becomes controlled and experimental, and it develops into an artificial instance of human interaction. When this kind of situation was created, the analyst engaged in engineering the patient's suggestibility instead of allowing him at least to participate in this quest for knowledge about his severely limited freedom. The analyst tended to work backwards from expected content to desired effect to technique, tailoring techniques to fit the requirements of the desired effect and then tailoring the effect to fit the preconceived notion. This made for the authoritarian dogmatism of Freud's psychoanalytic procedure in which the recall of the past was everything.

In hypnosis, the ideal recollection of the past required the complete absence of repetition; the personality organization embodying recurrent interpersonal patterns—the security operations and the distortions which emerged from them—was not a worthy area of inquiry in itself but only as a source of pathways to forgotten episodes. Beliefs which run much deeper in the fabric of personality than describing the oedipal period in sexual terms were not very important. They could easily be controlled by the dialetical interpretation and manipulation of the patient's positive transference—which the analyst might easily deny since he had also defined his role to the patient as being that of a mirror.

In Freud's view, the analyst practiced hypnotism in a new garb; he was only doing better what the hypnotherapist had always done. But though the old-style hypnotist often did oversimplify the road to recovery and appeal to fear and exaggerated dependency, he does not seem to have done it as systematically or as effectively as the psychoanalytic refinements now made possible. He did not have the dominating control of the sources of resistance which the psychoanalyst enjoyed; he did not have to create situations of reality to suit the postulates of an antecedent metapsychological theory, and he had to fit his technical activities to a reality which already existed. The psychoanalyst, on the other hand, followed the hypnotist in avoiding an ordinary serious interaction of two human beings to the end that the personality of one be reconstructed; he followed the hypnotist in not allowing transference distortions to emerge out of the free intercourse of two coequal human beings; he did not allow them simply to happen, but he found it necessary to effect them.

The fact is that certain transference distortions have qualities in common with post-hypnotic suggestion when a hypnotic situation is consciously structured or inadvertently created by the analyst. It should not blind us to the more important fact that certain transference phenomena cannot and will not occur in a hypnoid situation geared to engineering the patient's suggestibility; and the latter have very little in common with post-hypnotic suggestion. When the analytic situation is not structured expressly to evoke transference distortions from childhood, the analyst does not have to arrogate any unusual powers to himself; he expects to work with his patient in an open and uncircuitous way to arrive at a resolution of the patient's distortions. Thus, in contemporary psychoanalysis, we no longer look exclusively to the authoritarian attitude of the analyst to explain the distortion of him as an omnipotent god-like figure, though with some authoritarian analysts this may well be the case. Having abandoned the hypnotic picture of the analytic relationship, we are now in a position to look more carefully into the patient's current motivations for projecting divine beneficence onto the analyst. It is frequently found that he does not always idealize the analyst because he has internalized a parental imago but rather because the analyst does not fit into the patient's expectations from authorities which had been acquired not only in childhood but also in later relationships. By and large these past authority

figures have usually had a vested rather than an impartial interest in him, and he has had rare, if any, intimacies with any authority who had no personal stake in which way he decided to
construct his life.

It is historically true that Freud gave up the technique of hypnosis in the nineties on the strength of what he had learned from
Bernheim at the Nancy Clinic: that it was possible to force hypnotic subjects to recall what went on during a trance after they
had returned to their normal waking state.[10] It is also true that
as late as 1938 he found one of his best proofs for the reality of
unconscious processes in the post-hypnotic phenomena he had
observed at Bernheim's Clinic when he had originally studied
there in 1889.[11] There is a certain definite sense in which his
analogy is incontrovertible; it holds especially in so far as unconscious childhood perceptions and the attitudes which crystallized
out of them were evoked by an authoritarian analyst. But this
analogy has to be understood in the following context: Freud, it
will be recalled, did not give up suggestion in his last conception
of analytic technique but used it to counteract the transference
resistances—which are not similar to post-hypnotic suggestions
and do not come within the scope of this analogy. But he had
used suggestion to overcome what in his conception was also a
post-hypnotic kind of suggestion. The error in this therapeutic
thesis was that one could overcome something by reinforcing it
instead of analyzing it, that analytic therapy would require that
we foster the persistence of the very thing which caused the personal difficulty in the first place. Of course, Freud did not believe
that the system of resistances—the personality organization—was
the locus of difficulty; he believed that the repressed content was
the sole source which had to be tapped, a belief he had acquired
in hypnotherapeutic work.

In summary, Freud did not progress to the analysis of charac-

10 S. Freud, "Psychoanalysis," *Collected Papers*, Volume V, London: 1950,
pp. 110–111.
    11 S. Freud, "Some Lessons in Psychoanalysis," *Collected Papers*, Volume V,
London: 1950, p. 381, esp. fn. 1.

ter formation because his picture of the psychoanalytic situation had its roots in the hypnotist's relation to the patient; because his conception of unconscious processes did not transcend its origins in Bernheim's experiments with post-hypnotic suggestion; because his method of using suggestion did not differ significantly from hypnotic ways of using suggestion; because the technique of free association had its roots in the strict determination of post-hypnotic events; because his theory of dream interpretation was based on the central notion that unconscious sexual memories, like the forgotten hypnotic sources of post-hypnotic suggestion, have to be forced into awareness; and of course because his view of the analyst as a mirror was grounded in the mistaken idea that transferences, like post-hypnotic phenomena, will emerge only if the analyst has no perceptible or imperceptible influence on the patient's communications.

There is still the question about the general traits or defining qualities of transference distortion which distinguish it from open and direct experience. We can easily rely on technical rule-of-thumb procedures, as we often do in these matters, and allow society to tell students of psychopathology what sorts of behavior it will not tolerate at large. These socially defined deviations include that large mass of neglected human potential passing through the doors of our public and private institutions annually.

Since the psychoanalyst encounters what he calls distortions in his every-day practice, however, he finds it necessary to decide on the relative significance of various factors entering into their genesis and development. He has a multi-factor approach not simply to relieve his patients of anxiety, guilt or shame. This approach is dictated by the truth of the matter and not by any paternalistic motives. The idea that people become what they have a chance to become is at once a source of explanation of what they have become and a source of power to become what they desire and can still become. It is of course recognized that patients may use multi-factor concepts to defend themselves against the analysis of transference distortions and other disagreeable experiences by an appeal to cultural exigencies or physical disabilities. But multi-factor concepts are not surrendered on this account; instead they are used to facilitate an understanding and working through of the disagreeable experiences.

In explorations of personality, the validity of an interpretation which patients have placed on their experiences is not questioned even though it was based on distortion. Given the distortion, the interpretation was usually valid and the behavior which followed from it was essentially appropriate. Aside from this fact, there is of course the mutually expected eventuality that the patient will not always be prone to distort, and so, given the resolution of the distortion, he will probably be able to continue to make valid interpretations. It is essentially the operation of distortions, once defined, which is traced through the series of life-situations to the presenting difficulties, to the transference experiences encountered with the analyst. The interpretation of these life-situations is not wholly questionable—unless it could be demonstrated that the distortion has supplied all of the data for the patient's interpretation of his life-course. This is not ordinarily found in the private practice of psychoanalysis, and I do not suppose that even the most severely disturbed schizophrenic has misinterpreted or misjudged so much as he has misperceived and distorted certain aspects of those situations and felt constrained to overvalue them and allow them to outweigh other aspects.

This brings us to the chief point about distortion, and it is perhaps the most important one to be made about it. *As encountered in analytic therapy, it is a distortion in immediate experience rather than in judgment, interpretation or action*—the assumption being that clarifying the distorted perception will make for clearer judgment and so on. Locating the distortion in perception rather than in judgment or action will allow us to focus more sharply on the therapeutic issues. But what is perception? It is certainly dependent upon the proper operation of sensory organs and bodily musculature. Though neuro-physiological functions provide the perceptive process with some of its materials, it is hardly reducible to that kind of function. It is not reducible to neuro-physiology because it involves past feelings and attitudes, current strivings and sufferings, purposes and expectancies in the future. For during a distorted experience, one's current environment is misperceived through the intervention of perceptions which took place in previous communicational fields; it is a primed automatic response which overlooks distinctive characteristics in the current field, and it cannot be corrected simply by noting it or having it called to one's attention. Thus certain aspects of perceptual and communicational experience constitute a qualitatively unique domain of inquiry whose postulates may be translated into the language of physics and physiology but whose processes cannot be reduced to those of any other domain.

There is another possibly overriding reason for locating the process of distortion in perception. It throws into sharp relief the fact that we do not possess any single, inalienable principle of adjustment from which formulations of behavior are deducible. Imaginative potential cannot be prejudged; and the hitherto unexpressed ought not to be blotted out of human experience for the sake of a simplified theory of adjustment or a not so simple tool of repression during the analysis of transference. To be sure, the organization and development of personality are governed by the necessities of living through various modes of social thought and institutional conduct according to accidents of birth and biography. But this is not a process of simple acquiescence; it is not, moreover, a simple imposition of those patterns in psychoanalysis or life.[12] It is a cooperative process in which adequate working conceptions are molded out of a reciprocal modification of what one finds in his socio-cultural environment and what he brings to it. As ordinarily understood, "adjustment" is a superficial concept because it emphasizes the required end-products in social experience without acknowl-

[12] Even a cursory review of Freud's analysis of Dora reveals that one cannot impose a system of thought or behavior on another in order to "adjust" him to a preconceived notion of his circumstance. Most striking in this connection is that Dora was apparently not so dumb as to incorporate interpretations of her experience which did not accord with her own.

edging another distinct and perhaps conflicting factor as an integral phase of its process—a conscious effort to maintain and make felt in the experience of others that concrete increment of thoughts and attitudes which has developed out of one's past experience.

An enduring awareness of one's feelings, attitudes and judgments provides the best guide to that refined selective adjustment which lies between the Scylla of blind introjection of social standards and the Charybdis of adamant refusal to entertain them. Ideally, these phases of the process combine in ways which do justice to both. In the case of neurotics, they more or less do not; hence psychoanalysts must be open-minded with respect to varying personal organizations and the diverse styles of life which these variations imply. Psychoanalysts who are open-minded only in the sense that they are not openly critical may find their patients "adjusting"—renewing and repeating performances of social norms as if they were compulsive rituals. But they are not necessarily sympathetic students of human behavior who respect fundamental differences of motive and direction in personality organization. They do not see their patients adjusting in other equally respectable and perhaps more significant ways. This respect for motives is fundamental as a basis for personal adjustment, and if disturbed people do not find it in analytic therapy it is rather unlikely that they will be able to find it anywhere else.

Among the inalienable rights of man which we now take so much for granted that we do not take the trouble to spell them out, there stands the right to decide on the meaning of one's life. When patients, therefore, invite psychoanalysts to participate in this decision, it is not because they are fully alienated from this right. They have not yet surrendered their impulse to decide on the meaning of their lives. Instead, they may genuinely want to review and validate their perceptions and clarify their misperceptions; they may still reserve final judgment for themselves and we have no presumptive reason to believe otherwise.

chapter eight

Empirical Observations and an Operational Definition

ANALYSIS OF TRANSFERENCE is the major concern of the science and art of psychoanalysis. As a painter may be able to construct magnificent canvasses without delving into fine points of the physics of light and the science of color, so the psychoanalyst may be able to work through a therapeutic transference situation with little more than a cursory knowledge of psychological and psychoanalytic theories of personality development and disorder. It is dangerous to sever knowledge from action, and in so far as the analyst's anxieties permit him to have access to his mastery of theory and his therapeutic experience, his activities cannot be severed from these sources of skilled alertness and understanding during consultations. There are, however, no inviolable rules for the practical work, and this dictum is especially true about the ways and means of applying theoretical knowledge to transference material.

It may be laid down that all manifestations of distortion are reactive processes. Transference distortions and characterologic defenses are generically responses to the communication of others, however perceived. They are not active in type, and they are not genuine attempts at self-expression primarily designed to allow for the unhampered actions of others. For the analyst to respond directly to them in terms of their stipulated or implicit conditions would be rather ill conceived. The patient would certainly learn nothing from such responses to them because this is what they had earned for him in the past. Indeed, such earnings —the secondary gains—actually mobilize and reinforce them as personality trends rather than expose them to the light of analysis. They can be studied analytically with the patient so long as

he can see them as reactive phenomena but factually not in
direct reaction to the analyst's communications and relatedness
in the therapeutic process.

"Expectant libidinal impulses," Freud wrote, "will inevitably
be aroused by each new person coming upon the scene, and it is
more probable that both parts of the libido, the conscious and
the unconscious, will participate in this attitude." [1] In another
place, he stated unequivocally that the libidinal character of
transference is evident to anyone who has a true impression of
it. [2] Yet other workers have a true impression of the fact of transference and they do not support his view of its exclusively or
primarily libidinal character. The crucial question about Freud's
metapsychological theory of transference—whether libidinal impulses constitute it or whether it is a composite of reactions dis-
tilled out of specific encounters with some particular person or
persons in the patient's past in which much more than impulses,
libidinal or otherwise, are caught up—has already been discussed. Of even greater significance for therapeutic technique is
how we are to work with both the conscious and unconscious
"parts of the libido" in the transference relationship, since it is
the distorted and unconscious aspects of distortion which receive
most of our analytic attention. The conscious side—anxiety, per-
plexity, confusion, discomfort—is the staunch ally of the analyst
in attempts at collaborative exploration of its unconscious side.
If the unconscious side of a distortion continually monopolized
communication, the therapeutic aim would be not to explore
but to establish a beach-head in conscious attitudes which strive
to understand the distortion. [3] Where no such conscious desire
exists or can be reached, people do not ordinarily find their way

---

[1] S. Freud, "The Dynamics of Transference," *Collected Papers,* Volume II,
London: 1924, p. 313.

[2] S. Freud, *A General Introduction to Psychoanalysis,* Garden City: 1943,
p. 386.

[3] See S. Tower, "Management of Paranoid Trends in Treatment of a Post-
Psychotic Obsessional Condition," *Psychiatry,* X (1947), pp. 137–141. Also see,
below, *Addendum* (1964), p. 138.

to our consulting rooms, and if they request consultation because of external pressure, the therapeutic outlook is initially bleak. The beginning of conscious awareness of the operation of a transference distortion is thus the beginning of movement in analytic therapy, and should the conscious part of "the libido" also participate in it, we must maintain that the analyst is incapable of working with that particular patient or that he will have to investigate very seriously what the patient consciously ascribes to him. For when a distortion becomes conscious and retains this psychological status, the possibilities of analysis become dim indeed—witness a paranoid transformation and its blocking of therapeutic movement. But even such an eventuality does not necessarily rule out continued psychotherapeutic efforts.

That transference phenomena lie at the heart of the therapeutic process may sometimes be directly noted with or by the patient at various stages of treatment. Such statements are quite useless in themselves, however; the more effective way to communicate this fact is to demonstrate it by analytic work. At the outset, the patient usually has no idea of what is singularly significant in his communications. Careful and persistent therapeutic inquiry alone can convey the centrality of transference analysis to him. And there is no surer sign of therapeutic progress than his own detection of transference distortions; indeed every such observation requires some special sort of attention from the analyst. During every phase of analysis, there are significant transferences going on, and occasionally—especially at the early stages—neither analyst nor patient is aware of their larger significance. Despite the penetrating intuitive powers of some analysts, this significance, to be emotionally meaningful to the patient, must be painstakingly arrived at by joint inquiry. For if it springs full-blown from the head of Zeus, it can only be grasped by one who has divine attributes. Even if the therapeutic relationship is a good one, nothing need necessarily happen to the firm personality trends of the patient in spite of the apparent correctness of the interpretations—except perhaps to reinforce resistance and mobilize defenses. Through the pressure of unconstructive experience, the analyst who possesses remarkable intuitive facility will eventually develop skilled restraint about his interpretive contributions.

All transference distortions are not equally crucial for the outcome of therapy. The general distinction between distorted and non-distorted experiences must of course be kept in mind throughout the analytic process. It is often impossible for the analyst to know at the beginning which is specifically which and what its meaningful context is. These distinctions are tentatively arrived at as the analysis progresses, and they are always subject to reconstruction with the appearance of new facts. In addition to this general distinction, there is the need to decide on the relative significance of the various distortions in each individual case. There are no fixed rules for deciding in advance on this matter, because some analysts are capable of working much more intuitively than others. Besides, the live significance of data depends on two very different kinds of factors: The selection of crucial facts which have been observed and arranged to delineate the central difficulties must be graphic and compelling; and the urgency of this interpretation at a particular therapeutic stage involves the patient's readiness to discern the incongruity of his distortion when set off against a more syntaxic interpretation of the facts.

There are at least three sorts of transference manifestations which may be distinguished. Those that are therapeutically neutral have no immediate relevance to the analytic process at a given point and are to that extent ignored; those defenses against an insight whose underlying anxiety calls for the analyst's active intervention; and those that reflect long-standing interpersonal distortions, entrenched and crystallized in typical interactions, require the active collaboration of both analyst and patient. Usually it is a resistance that accompanies the second and third types of transference manifestations. In the second, it is usually necessary to look into therapeutic contexts of the immediate present or recent past; and when it is a central interpersonal attitude, a graphic picture of the patient's personal functioning is usually necessary.

It is clearly impossible to classify transferences in a way that will be completely satisfactory. Some may find it more congenial to think in terms of constructive and destructive distortions; yet this value-judgment is not always what the patient will find most conducive to the analysis of the constituent factors that set a specific defensive operation in motion. But whether one makes his classification in genetic terms, value terms or operationally, there is a serious drawback to this whole business of classification. While some scientific categories fit life better than others, all of life cannot be squeezed into scientific categories. Thus, communications that are therapeutically neutral in one context may be crucial in another; those treated as immediate defensive operations in one context may eventually reveal themselves to be long-standing interpersonal distortions; and with these shifts in therapeutic context different logical distinctions are indicated.

Therapeutic probings of intolerable feelings or thoughts which the patient has never felt free to divulge to another person usually call forth a distorted reaction. This is what Freud called resistance and Sullivan referred to as a security operation, the intervention of the self-system to modify anxiety; the latter is an operational definition that describes what the process does. Resistance is a crude concept because it implies that the patient is actually resisting the analyst's line of inquiry. In his final statement, Freud had developed his theory of transference analysis on this basis and held that it had to be overcome. The analyst may experience it in this way, and when he does, it is time for him to undertake an investigation of his own unconscious attitudes toward the patient. For what has been called resistance is the patient's defense against processes he learned to consider unacceptable. He avoids the clarification of his distortions because of the fear, shame, guilt or powerlessness that once accompanied the unacceptable feelings when they were direct responses and had objective reference, and so he resists reactively as if the analyst personified those other people who provoked the intolerable experiences. The patient actually dislikes these intolerable thoughts and painful feelings; he is not going to revive and reexperience them if he can help it; so he gets in his own way, stops the flow of his communication—resists himself as it were—and introduces new barriers into the therapeutic relationship.

To my knowledge, there is no way to eliminate these obstructions but by continuing experience with a friendly person who has an open mind about things which make the patient judge himself harshly. If he does not want to see what is being kept out of awareness, the analyst has no direct way of hearing it. The interpretation of dreams and like phenomena can at best provide circuitous approximations that may reassure both the patient and the analyst that something is known, but this does not reveal the plethora of intimate and highly individual detail which has not been discussed. The patient may eventually see that there is more to be gained by looking into what can hardly be so irrational, painful or whatever he ascribes to it, that the difficulties which brought him to treatment are still with him and will most likely remain with him if he does not say what comes to his mind, and that since he cannot, in his present state, judge what is useful in the analytic enterprise, he is actually preventing further collaboration of a possibly fruitful sort by withholding significant facts about himself.

In analytic therapy, defensive distortions can be touched off by practically anything the analyst is, says or does. But they are already ongoing affairs before the therapeutic interaction takes place. A comment or question may point to areas which the patient has repressed over so long a period of time that he is now incapable of investigating them. Further attempts at inquiry are seen as a violation of individual sanctity. The analyst is perceived as having all sorts of intentions, as being inimical, pressuring, prodding, sarcastic, scornful, helpful, interested, parental, loving: he is construed as a protector or an antagonist ambivalently concerned with his patient's needs and as requiring a host of other things which have or had meaning in integrations with people other than the analyst. Of course, the information called for is not readily available to the patient. But the striking fact is that he cannot stop and reflect upon the question. Everything but the information called for by the question comes to the fore. Communication has been cut off in one direction and proceeds in another, and the patient's need to avoid anxiety has been transformed into a transference distortion.

These distorted constructions have a telescopic quality. In a sense, they are open at both ends and point in two directions, since the patient's articulated defenses against the analyst are usually the same as his defenses against his own anxiety and insight. As the analytic relationship moves to closer quarters, the patient begins to experience things in a more constricted fashion, and these perceptions of the analyst can only be deflected from his distortions of himself. It may be compared to the painter who has a dozen colors on his palette and finds himself using shades of only one or two for reasons he does not know.

The original experiences and the repressed facts cannot be entirely recovered in their original form. They are reconstructed piecemeal from the evidence of specific transference manifestations. If we demand their full recovery, our patients may, as Freud discovered, supply them in a fantastic form. In fact, one may question whether reconstruction of the forgotten events whose effects are repeated in transference experiences is the kernel of the therapeutic action of analysis or whether the repeated testing of their effects enlightens the patient. Our patient does not know the original or repressed phenomena; we do not know them either. After a few months of collaborative endeavor, we may learn some effects of these postulated events or situations, and so we can put our observations and inferences at his disposal. When confronted with knowledge about the communicated effects of those difficulties, he may or may not assimilate it. At first he usually does not, and this is the action of security operations which later evolve into transference distortions. But if the analyst's observations are valid and his inferences warranted, and if the analytic situation is not botched so that the transference is turned into a real situation where the analyst actually does what the patient, in terms of his own distorted personification, anticipated that he would do, more information is usually obtained which throws light on the distorted aspects of these interpersonal involvements.

The emotional nuances of past difficulties which are drawn out in long-standing relationships will not be recalled in their entirety. But their effects, as experienced in the present and affecting the future life-course, are at least vaguely apparent to the patient in some ways in his everyday life. And they are undeniable when he can experience them openly with the analyst. That they are undeniable in therapeutic transference situations is of the utmost importance. It means that the therapeutic situation is ultimately the psychological learning situation. It means that the cooperative observation of these effects with a skilled person makes defensive obfuscation useless at best. And it means that precision in discerning and delineating the pattern of the distortion spells success or failure in the therapeutic situation. In view of this fact, the description of distorted perceptions has to be evolved gradually, tentatively and provisionally.

Other reasons may be forwarded: psychoanalysts have long since recognized the futility of perpetuating the myth of omnipotence or omniscience; they no longer foster the myth that mind-reading is possible; and philosophers of science now take for granted the idea that knowledge is to be arrived at inferentially and that empirical inquiry is specific in character. But in terms of the subject matter and aims of psychoanalytic therapy, any persistent lack of preciseness in describing what goes on in the "me-you" distortion will convince the patient that the analyst lacks understanding, fails to hear him or perhaps more simply that he is a fool.

The analysis of distortions of people outside the therapeutic situations often lacks psychological immediacy. Since a patient could not possibly have told the whole story in a session or even a year, he can produce new data that usually provide him with satisfactory defenses against an interpretation. He can describe situations in which this interpretation does not entirely hold, or raise questions about the importance of other factors involved or about their relative weight. So far as the future course of the analysis is concerned, it is safer to be wrong about such extra-analytic situations because patients know that the analyst was not at the reported situation and was actually in no position to observe all of the data at first hand. But the evaluation of the distortion of the analyst has to approximate the truth of the situation rather closely, the maxim being to "strike when the iron is hot."

Whether it is always necessary to include historical material in a mutative interpretation is a moot question so far as the therapeutic side of the matter is concerned. The most effective interpretations of transference distortions are those which point up "here and now" experiences, those which lay bare the patient's immediate experiences of the analyst. These interpretations must be made with extreme care. They need be no more than a question or a non-verbal gesture, but an error can lead to needless complication during the treatment. They are very difficult to evade when they are accurate because the patient is presented with the evidence while he is in the throes of an immediate experience.

During the expression of distortions, the patient may also ascribe characteristics to the analyst which the analyst would ordinarily acknowledge as valid without hesitation. These expressions are not always to be taken at face value, however. Before such an acknowledgement is made, the attitudinal context and feeling-tone of the communication are to be considered, for they are as noteworthy as its verbal content. The analyst's excessive readiness to acknowledge his real traits may prove to be the undoing of the analytic inquiry. The prima facie fact is that the patient has come for an exploration of his own personality. It is still his own psychoanalysis and he may rightly be perturbed by the analyst's readiness to respond to the cognitive content of his remarks. An early responsiveness to such observations about the analyst can certainly impede the analytic process. In fact, there are times when the patient does not really want to hear that his descriptions of the analyst are true; he may be intent on communicating his attitude or feeling-tone, his defensive love or hostility, or simply trying to reassure himself for whatever purpose. Because the patient is primarily interested in his own analysis, it is incumbent upon the analyst to look for the defensive quality of these accurate descriptions. At certain stages of the analysis, we have no alternative but to attribute a defensive quality to them. If they do not have this defensive quality, we must at least wonder about the need they satisfy for the patient; for he certainly does not consult us to analyze our personalities. It is often observed that this structuring of the analytic situation satisfied the patient's need to see just how the analyst can fall into his personal scheme of distortions just as he usually seeks out other people for this end. And when this is attempted with the analyst, it serves the same purpose as it usually does with others—to avoid looking through his own distortions and facing himself.

This may not always seem to be true. In the case of detached and withdrawn people who make feeble efforts to reach out to others, an open acceptance of accurate descriptions may convey to them that the analyst is interested in their observations about people, interested enough to accept valid judgments about himself. This may not only facilitate their productivity and improve the therapeutic relationship; it may also encourage them to express and seriously consider their own as well as the analyst's observations. It must be noted even here, however, that the response is not necessarily or solely to the cognitive content of their remarks. It is again a response to the attitudinal and feeling context of the therapeutic situation.

There are still other exceptions to the above comments, the most important being at the terminating phases of the psychoanalytic procedure. One probable sign that an analysis is nearing completion is the patient's general perception of the analyst as a real person. But it has to be evaluated as part of the total clinical picture; it cannot be understood in isolation. This is a probable sign of completion on the view that we see others as we see ourselves: When the patient can see the analyst as a real person it may be presumed that he can also see himself as a real person. Operationally, this is how the analyst may obtain irrefutable evidence that the patient's distortions have been worked through. For in working through to a valid picture of the analyst as a person, he will have to realize, in the course of it, that interferences with his growth and development can be mastered in his relations with another person. And mastery is signified by objective perceptions—objective in the sense that at least two observers can describe them in the same way.

When transference distortions are conscious or close enough to conscious awareness to be brought into focus by the analyst's comments, this therapeutic effort often succeeds. However, it usually cannot work when they are unconscious. These interfering attitudes that prevent the pursuit of his problems are as inaccessible as the problems themselves, and mere suggestion or mere clarification will not effect any changes. The analysis of security operations is indicated because they obstruct the patient's use of his own resources for coping with his problems. This makes sense in the following type of paradigm: When the patient initially experienced his difficulties, he repressed them because they were painful, shameful and so on. The subsequent series of situations through which he moved held the possibilities for both repetition and clarification of the fact that his experiences with a particular person were undergone with that person at certain definite times and not necessarily connected with all people at all times. But he was not open to corrective influence. Over a long period of time and through a variety of situations, defenses against repetition became more important than openness to new experience. Potentialities remain dormant until a new experience with an understanding person makes it possible for those originally unacceptable feelings to be felt and others to develop.

The quintessence of analysis is this repetition of distortions and anxieties under new conditions. Repetition is the clue to the establishment of an unconscious defensive attitude and repetition is the clue to its dissolution. The patient continually tests his self-concept with the analyst; he continually communicates his distortions of the analyst. Those aspects of the perception which are acknowledgeable as valid cannot be analyzed, while its other presumably distorted aspects are repeatedly subjected to the test of interpersonal experience. He may finally surrender a distortion because it has no basis in the shared experience in the psychoanalytic situation. He may at first speak without understanding what he says, and through continual repetition, finally begin to hear himself; this constitutes the break-through where the attitude is seen to be the invalid one that it is. By undergoing an experience under novel conditions with a person who can acknowledge the truth when he sees it, the patient may finally develop to the point where he can openly acknowledge the truth about himself. This is an essential ingredient of any genuine sort of personality reconstruction, for here the patient learns that distortions are distortions.

Strictly speaking, this repetition under novel conditions is not really repetition at all but a very novel experience. Therapeutic transference is thus the opposite of repetition-compulsion—a mechanistic concept at best because while emphasizing frequencies in behavior it did not take the potentialities of plasticity and growth into account. Unlike the so-called transferences of everyday life, therapeutic transference holds the promise of breaking through to an understanding of the compulsion. If one insists, it may be considered an actual instance of the repetition-compulsion; but it is also and chiefly a potential negation of it.

The evidences of transference distortions provide clues to the fact that the patient is anxiously and defensively involved with the analyst. They include situations in which vocal communication, communication by gesture and bodily movements, and transitory somatic symptoms during the course of analysis are important media of distorted processes. The pitch and tonal quality of voice are sources of leads which may turn out to be just as significant as the actual content of verbal communication. This means that the patient can control his voice pitch much less effectively than the content of his verbalizations; his verbal communication of a distortion depends on the organization of the "economic-dynamic" factors in the therapeutic relationship, and so, once expressed, it frequently loses its immediacy as impulse or feeling and is dissipated in hesitation—that it is irrational, silly, ridiculous or "I know it makes no sense but . . ."

The following is a partial list of situations which usually indicate an experience of the analyst in terms of a personification:

(1) The patient expresses an unreasoning dislike for the analyst.

(2) The patient describes the analyst as unreal, mechanical or depersonalized. When the analyst makes a comment or asks a question designed to gather more information, the patient tends to ignore its point while seeming to respond to it.

(3) The patient becomes overinvolved with some personal trait of the analyst that has little if any bearing on his experience or skill—or even on the patient's ability to work with him.

(4) The patient expresses excessive liking for the analyst, feels he is the best or only possible analyst for him, and claims that no one else in the world could assume and successfully carry out the therapeutic task.

(5) The patient dreads the hours with the analyst and is persistently uncomfortable during them.

(6) The patient is preoccupied with the analyst to an unusual degree in the intervals between sessions and may find himself imagining remarks, questions or situations involving the analyst. The analyst may appear in the patient's dreams as himself.

(7) The patient finds it difficult to focus on any aspect of his problems. He is vague about them and discusses them as if he were consulting the analyst about his case as one professional colleague to another.

(8) The patient is habitually late for appointments or shows other disturbances about time arrangements, such as running over the end of the hour or saying that he does not want to leave. Any disturbance about any aspect of the arrangements, once entered upon and mutually agreed upon, fall into this category.

(9) The patient continually argues, seeks love, remains uninvolved or indifferent about important problems in his life—in fact, continually does any one sort of thing in an automatic way.

(10) The patient becomes defensive with the analyst and exhibits extreme vulnerability to the analyst's observations, inferences or interpretations.

(11) The patient consistently misunderstands or persistently requires further clarification of the analyst's interpretations. When he never agrees with them, this transference process can be tested simply by repeating to the patient an observation of his own which he had made earlier in the hour—and he will usually disagree with that too.

(12) The patient seeks to elicit a particular emotional response from the analyst—for instance, by provocative remarks, double-edged questions or dramatic statements.

(13) The patient becomes overconcerned with the confidentiality of his work with the analyst.

(14) The patient beseechingly or angrily looks for sympathy regarding some sort of maltreatment, real or imagined, at the hand of some authority figure.

(15) The patient habitually introduces sessions in a characteristic way—with a certain kind of question, a series of alternative topics for discussion or a series of gestures.

(16) The patient praises the analyst for improvements in his life which are actually not direct results of psychoanalytic therapy.

(17) The patient expresses the desire to be the only patient of his analyst.

(18) The patient takes a leading question of the analyst, re-phrases it in the form of a declarative statement and considers this adequate—that is, instead of following its lead into history or some current problem.

(19) The patient's facial expression and voice pitch change markedly, not necessarily in congruence with the apparent meaning of his verbalizations—for example, specific tics, uncontrolled fits of laughter and crying.

(20) The patient changes his bodily position in characteristic ways whether he is seated or lying on the couch—for example, a turn of the head, an uncontrolled ("nervous") movement of the legs, a crossing and uncrossing of the legs or arms.

(21) The patient reports transitory physical symptoms during treatment. They may be evident only during the analytic situa-

tion or they may be reported as accentuated or newly observed in relation to other people.

Therapeutic attempts to explore any of these experiences usually run into the anxiety which any move to act otherwise entails for the patient. They will touch off the feelings of being uncomfortable, exposed, tense, threatened or the pressing need to get away from the issue at hand. This is why it is so difficult to explore them directly. Such head-on explorations develop into subtle and even overt struggles for power in the analytic situation, or they may become diffuse in intellectual discussions that go in the opposite direction of feeling experience; and either way, new difficulties may actually be produced which will have to be analyzed. Nevertheless, the other alternative—to overlook the anxiety accompanying transference manifestations—is an even more barren tack for analytic therapy to take. To circumvent this anxiety would make the analyst a partner to the defense against anxiety and serve only to reinforce the repetitive transference pattern. Because he did not see it as a reactive process designed especially to avoid or assuage anxiety, he was not able to elucidate its essential purpose in the "me-you" relationship, and since the patient would just as soon not see it either, a significant occasion for intensive analysis will have passed unnoticed. Interpersonal skill, tact, alertness and sensitivity are required of the analyst to avoid the futility of a power-struggle without endangering the possibilities which every such transference manifestation presents for the intensification of the analytic process.

An operational definition may now be set forth which generalizes these enumerated observations: *When, in the patient-analyst relationship, the patient's anxiety is aroused and interferes with continued collaborative endeavor on the problem at hand, the alteration of the patient's behavior, verbal or otherwise, is a transference distortion, the emergence of a parataxic communication in the therapeutic situation.* It is important to note that Freud did not consider the problem of anxiety in any of his writings on the transference phenomenon, and there is no reference to transference in his significant work on anxiety in 1926. The rela-

tionship between the two may be inferred from his concept of
the early traumatic experience. But this dialectical exercise is
fraught with insuperable difficulties. For even in the formulation
of 1926, he conceived of anxiety as attached to the symptomatic
conflict and there was no explicit change in therapeutic goal;
suggestion was to be utilized in the form of transference, resistances were to be overcome with the aid of suggestion, and his aim
was still the hypnotic one of remembering the original trauma.

Therapeutic transference, as operationally defined, refers specifically to observed parataxic distortions of communication and
relatedness. The transference does not exist as a process. A number of specific occasions to which this concept refers does exist,
and it is these occasions we study. The varieties of communicated nuances from one occasion to another denotes specific differences in the transference. They reveal whether it is related to a
parent in infancy or childhood, a chum in pre-adolescence, a
sibling in any of these periods, or a companion in that extended
struggle for maturity called adolescence; and these differences
also provide clues to the type of experience out of which the
distortion emerged. Perceiving the analyst in accordance with
any one of these personified images signifies the experience of
anxiety among other things—an unfounded fear that is followed
by an expectation of something or other from the analyst. It is
important to keep tabs on the context as well as the content of
the distortion, lest the present experience be rewarded with
continued ignorance. But there is no way of avoiding such therapeutic experiences, if the meaning of anxiety and defensive operations is our goal.

[*Addendum* (1964): More extensive clinical material, beyond the listing of
observations of transference, is in B. Wolstein, *Freedom to Experience*, New
York: 1964, where the attempt is made to place them in the context of an
ongoing psychoanalytic experience, in addition to their context of the general
structure of psychoanalytic inquiry. See, especially, Chapter II, for an interpretation of resistance as a function of transference, and Part Two, for the
relativity of transference and countertransference, anxiety and distortion in
reconstructive experience, and unconscious aspects of the immediate present.
In B. Wolstein, *Countertransference*, New York: 1959, Chapter IV, are some
varieties of psychoanalytic experience that are directly a function of the
analyst's personality.]

chapter nine

Freedom in Transference and Metapsychology

I DOUBT WHETHER ANYONE will take issue with the proposition that transference distortions constitute a serious curtailment of psychological freedom. But I also doubt that its implications have been fully realized in current views of transference analysis. Freud's conception was hypnotically oriented, and because the resulting technique was authoritarian, few analyses were carried through to the point where the patient was capable of making his own analyses of his transferences. One may define psychological freedom as an absence of restraint or as self-determination within the context of one's social and personal conditions of life. But irrespective of how it is defined, it cannot be achieved in psychoanalysis when analysts find it necessary to accommodate the distortions of their patients rather than understand why those accommodated conditions emerged in the first place.

A very peculiar state of affairs arises when anxieties are accommodated; for these accommodations develop into a spiral effect in which they are in turn reacted to by the patient, to which reactions the analyst responds, to which reactions the patient responds and so on without the initial accommodation being inquired into in order to see how the problems of the one participant had interlocked with the problems of the other. If the analyst finds it necessary to accommodate the defensive system of the patient in order to keep the work on a smooth course, the therapy will be headed for rough going. Both the analyst and the patient will eventually reach a point where they will want to know what they are trying to accomplish, and neither may have any positive ideas about it. This nexus of interpersonal processes is usually beyond the awareness of both participants, since the analytic therapy has been structured to satisfy their needs for security; but the patient derives very little, if any, benefits from it. Whichever the analyst feels on principle to be the road to good analysis—focus on present experiences, past events or future anticipations, he may unsuspectingly conform with the patient's established security operations. And this does not augur well for the therapeutic outcome, not only because the patient's transference distortions have encountered a customary impasse, although this in itself is unfortunate enough, but chiefly because they have become enmeshed with the analyst's distortions or blind-spots. Neither participant enjoys the psychological freedom necessary to come to grips with the deadlock in the interaction. The analyst may feel motivated to obscure or halt the workings of his distortion as he usually does in any relationship, but his derivative defenses will only move the patient away from that particular center of anxiety. The patient may sense the complexity of this reaction in the characteristic way in which he has sensed the unconscious motives of others in the past. In fact, important therapeutic clues might be derived from the way a patient reacts to someone else's distortions once he recognizes their presence. The unfortunate thing in this turn of events is that the analyst, when burdened with his own misperceptions, cannot direct his attention to the patient's reactions; he can only wait and see.[1] If, on the other hand, the analyst has a firm awareness of his past distortions and can estimate his contribution to this parataxic interlocking of personality patterns, it need not necessarily lead to total therapeutic loss. When such occasions are skillfully analyzed, they can in fact lead to mutual psychological benefit. The interaction has been live, crucial and meaningful. But it must be emphasized that the analyst must have at least a modicum of understanding of the probable effects he can have on people and some estimate of their probable reactions to him.

When the patient has suffered enough discontent to have prompted him to undertake analysis, the analyst would be remiss

[1] C. Thompson, R. M. Crowley and E. S. Tauber, "Symposium on Counter-Transference," *Samiksa*, VI (1952), pp. 205–228.

in the task which he has undertaken if he failed to provide an integrated conception of what he had heard which would point in the direction of further constructive collaboration. By conveying a definition of the problem as he sees it, he is also letting the patient know he understands that there is a real problem to be resolved. If he does this from the very outset instead of making genetic interpretations which are so easily incorporated by the patient's defensive system, he actually reinforces the original insight with a firmer conception of the problem. The groundwork for the ensuing collaboration with the patient is laid by arriving at a common understanding of the difficulty, even if this understanding is not the most pleasant for him to hear. When this sort of active collaboration does not take place, the analysis will bog down in the labyrinth of the patient's security operations—only this time they will have been aided and abetted by the analyst's. And this is the way his constructive efforts had bogged down in his interactions with other people prior to entering analysis.

Once this interlocking of experience takes place, the possibilities for therapeutic movement are very slim unless the analyst is willing and able to inspect his own personal characteristics which intertwine with the patient's troubled system of security operations. Without such a self-examination he will be of very little help to the patient. And he would even be helpless with himself if he were faced with similar circumstances. If he does occasionally prove helpful under these conditions, he will not know what he does that helps. The patient will have lost an opportunity to learn about his distortions and his ways of dealing with them. In effect, the analyst will be duplicating the error of Freud's formulation in the *Introductory Lectures* where positive transference was utilized instead of analyzed. This state of affairs usually gets the analytic process into a rut or, as it has been euphemistically referred to, a plateau. For the analytic possibilities are negligible just because the analyst cannot call significant aspects of this interlocking of interpersonal processes to the patient's attention.

The extent to which an analyst is able to stay with his patient's distortions of him will govern the extent to which they can be experienced in his presence. His ability to observe and describe them with detached non-reciprocating interest will condition his patient's opportunity to hear himself. It will allow for their repetition until the anxiety and mechanical defensiveness cannot escape the awareness of either participant. We do not gear our work simply to the disintegration of habitually distorted perceptions, however. Habit, as Nietzsche once put it, is the staff of life; it confers organization, meaning and continuity on human experience. We work with our patients to make freedom and flexibility in habit-formation possible, and we adapt our skills to the individuality of each particular patient.

These days when so many of our patients have quite a lot of sophistication about the concepts and operations of psychoanalysis as reported in the literature, it frequently happens that an analysis which falls into the customary and expected routine is not really an analysis at all. The analyst thinks he is trying to help—which he may sincerely be doing without recognizing his inutility—and the patient conducts himself as if he were in analysis. These sophisticated patients disguise their extreme dependency with the conscious idea that they are really the best judges of their interpersonal processes. But their competitiveness is not quite as disguised as their dependency; they would like the analyst to "supervise" their analyses of themselves rather than make the raw data accessible to the analyst. The customary analytic routine will not work especially if it falls into a frame of reference which the patient thinks the analyst accepts. And this is also true for those patients who have acquired a parlor knowledge of Freud's views and expect every analyst to subscribe to them; they tend to act out a pseudo-experience of transference-love and oversexualize all of their communications because this is the way they expect to be "cured."

For example, a patient once attempted to fulfill the requisites of the mature personality as defined by some of the thinkers who taught at the psychoanalytic training center with which I am associated. It was later learned that this constituted an acting out of what he thought was acceptable in fulfillment of the requirements for successful analysis; and of course I was not supposed to be interested in his sexual difficulties because the study of interpersonal relations somehow did not include this most intimate of relationships as he saw it. There was little that could be done until this was discovered, but on discovery it became even more difficult to get at the centers of his anxiety. In this instance, a set of symptoms was temporarily relieved by suggestions which were never directly made to the patient but were implied by what he knew about the analyst. It was suggestion nonetheless which had to be dealt with as if it were actually made by the analyst. The analysis of defensive operations had yet to be accomplished, even though it now became harder to get at them. On analysis, it turned out that the patient had disguised his symptoms and was actually arranging his psychological situation so that he would not have to resolve his transference problems. This became the topic for further analysis, and if it had not been inadvertently discovered, the analysis might have had a fruitless ending. It had yet to begin in a genuine sense, for his anxieties had become somewhat further removed from awareness, and another sort of defense engendered in the analytic interaction had to be worked through before the analysis could be resumed in earnest.

This experience raised some questions about Freud's concept of transference neurosis. He once had noted that the patient's illness grew continuously like any living thing.[2] This observation is essentially valid, and it not only casts serious doubt on his earlier studies of infantile neuroses in themselves; it also opens to question all theories of transference analysis that sever the therapeutic situation from previous and concurrent experience. The very notion of a transference neurosis having to be created for productive analysis, however, separates two of Freud's basic points of view—the dynamic and the genetic. To separate transference phenomena from other situations in which the unconscious distortions originally got their start or in which they were later reinforced actually misses the utility of analytic therapy; to hold

2 S. Freud, *A General Introduction to Psychoanalysis*, Garden City: 1943, p. 386.

with Freud that we have to deal with a newly created and transformed neurosis [3] would overlook the cumulative and continuous
character of distortions in psychotherapy and life even if it emphasized the final "battlefield" on which the therapeutic aim is
accomplished. This emphasis is essentially correct, but it does not
require that we view the patient's transference experiences as a
neurotic transformation of the central distortions which made it
necessary for him to seek treatment in the first place.

The obstacles to accepting this idea that a transference neurosis
be created go much deeper than theoretic contradiction. They
arise directly in the therapeutic situation: for little is actually
gained other than increased resistance to pursuing the character
problems when the patient repeats an earlier distorted experience
with the analyst to the end that his symptoms be beneficently
resolved and the analyst reciprocates in terms of these transference conditions. The neurosis actually develops again with the
analyst as a reacting participant, and the possibilities for analytic benefit diminish of course. An extremely skilled approach to
this situation is required of the analyst for therapeutic movement
to take place, but it is extremely unlikely that he will be able to
do this since he could not originally maintain himself as a participant observer and was compelled to contribute to the development of the transference neurosis.

We do not seek a therapeutic situation where we have to deal
with a newly created neurosis which has replaced an earlier one.
The distortions were operant before the contact with the analyst,
and they are still operant in the same way even though they may
now be studied microscopically in collaboration with the analyst.
The therapeutic transference situation provides the patient with
a psychological microscope, so that he can now inspect his distortions more closely than he ever could before. Encountering another person, his personality structure begins to function as usual.
The chief difference is that this time it will function in reaction
to a skilled person who will not—it is hoped—respond in terms
of the distortion but rather in ways to point out the nature of the

[3] Reference footnote 2, p. 386.

distortion. Thus the therapeutic transference is a truly novel experience for the patient—not as a repetition of distortions but as an opportunity to observe and understand them. And the concept of transference neurosis is a misnomer at best, since the therapeutic transference situation is instituted to understand distortions in interpersonal relations at large as well as in relation to the analyst.

As is usually the case with Freud's observations, it was entirely correct to describe a transference neurosis under the conditions of his method for analytic therapy. His technique was geared to overcoming the character resistances in order to resolve the presented symptoms; being symptom-oriented it was bound to foster the creation of the character neurosis anew, for the method did not consider the total personality analytically. To be sure, the patient wanted relief from the oppression of his symptoms, but because this relief was provided without his acquiring a firm understanding of why they came into being, he developed his neurotic attachments to the analyst. Now it is possible to work with symptoms and character problems together in such a way that there will be an interplay between the very evident anxiety about the symptoms and much less evident anxieties about the character problems. Out of this interplay may emerge that desirable situation in which the symptoms will be taken care of by the patient while the character problems of which they are symptomatic will become the chief topic of inquiry. By and large, the analyst's own concerns about the gravity of the symptom will determine what he will be able to do about it. But his concern about working with it to the exclusion of character problems may become more important than his evaluation of the symptom; and this may turn out to be more difficult for the analyst to deal with than his concern about the persistence of the symptom.

We are always faced with making a decision on the relative importance of symptom and character trait in every therapeutic undertaking; we have to decide whether we will consider the conflict in traits the subject of analysis or whether we will work toward the resolution of symptoms as presented by the patient.

This decision is usually arrived at with the patient through an impressionistic estimation of his goals in treatment. To put the matter in this way does not determine the actualities of any specific therapeutic interaction, for apart from the patient's own estimate of his treatment goals and future potentialities, there is always the analyst's operational approach to be considered—a fact which might be brought to the patient's attention more frequently.

This distinction between presenting symptom and character problem is, on the face of it, a rather prosaic one. But it enables us to differentiate radically between two types of therapeutic approach, between a direct approach to the presented content of the problem and an approach to the function of the problem in the total personality. The one enters directly into the weighing of the various factors which constitute the neurotic symptoms; the other does as little as possible with the neurotic symptoms itself and focusses on the personality trends which set them in motion. The one is reminiscent of the early hypnotic and suggestive psychotherapies which Freud had partially abandoned in the nineties; by proceeding straightaway to the patient's construction of his symptom, the therapist automatically ignored the personality disorder of which it was symptomatic. The other also takes the presenting conflicts as symptoms, but symptoms which are to be studied indirectly.

Since any thoroughgoing analysis of a symptom involves a successful resolution of the personality difficulties of which it is symptomatic, this distinction may only reflect a difference in starting point for investigation. However, the chief shortcoming of the symptomatic approach is that once the patient achieves a satisfactory resolution of his conflict he no longer has interest in going any further with his analysis. Of course, he may want to continue the reworking of his personality structure on his own, and that is all right too.

By and large, this distinction cannot be rigidly adhered to in actual practice. The character analyst must occasionally comment on the conflictual factors that immediately trouble the patient, and the suggestive therapist cannot resolve the conflict for the patient in his everyday life; the patient has to do something for himself. Furthermore, if the presenting problem is thoroughly studied and actually alleviated, some concomitant character change can be expected to have taken place; and conversely, any successful analysis of character problems leads to the satisfactory resolution of the presenting conflict. Though this distinction may not always be of central significance, every analyst must decide whether he will concentrate on the symptoms or the character problems in the study of his patient's communications.

Aside from the personal predilections of any particular therapist, there are certain advantages in the character-analytic point of view. It does not require moral exhortations of the analyst. It does not put him in the position of having to judge a single alternative course of action to be better or worse than any other of a series of conflicting alternatives. It leaves the patient with a sense of his own prerogative in making judgments of value, for the analyst contributes to psychological freedom and initiative by helping him to acquire information about his characteristic patterns of functioning without entering into his final judgment. This does not mean that the science of psychoanalysis is value-free; it definitely is not. But it does mean that there is a difference between understanding and judgment, that the patient may make his own affirmative judgments based on understanding his psychodynamics among other things and that the therapist cannot interfere with the value-affirmations of his patients even when they run counter to his "better" judgment.

Finally, this point of view relieves the analyst of the impossible burden of omniscience and deprives him of any claim to it. In so doing, it allows the patient the elbow-room he needs to investigate his own quest for an omniscient figure. By focussing on function rather than content, the psychoanalyst tacitly admits his inability to deal competently with every sort of content his patients may encounter—legal, ethical, educational, vocational, social, political, economic, ideological, neuro-physiological, gastrointestinal and a thousand and one other things. No analyst can possibly be proficient in every specialty; he cannot have expert knowledge about all of the things a person can possibly encounter; and if he introduces his commonsense view of things, he must assume that his is better than the patient's. On the other hand, if he can offer competent opinions on matters the patient discusses which are beyond the domain of interpersonal processes, it is probably best for him to offer them sparingly. The character analyst tries to place at the disposal of his patients a secure understanding of their transference processes so that they can make their own judgments of value in life. He assumes that he is being consulted as a specialist in psychological matters and willingly offers opinions in his own field of expertness when they are indicated. But he does not assume, as a psychotherapeutic specialist, that he is being consulted for information about education, sociology, the law or even about the nervous system and gastrointestinal disorders. In fact, where the psychoanalyst happens to have competence in any of these fields, his patients may try to use it in a defensive way by having him discuss anything but their psychological difficulties even though he is being consulted for his knowledge about psychological difficulties.

It cannot be denied that the personality of each analyst will require certain emphasis in technique which other analysts will be able to do without. How each analyst will use psychoanalytic knowledge cannot be laid down in an arbitrary blueprint, and so psychoanalysis, like any other science, is ultimately an art. An attempt at therapeutic intervention succeeds only if it is in line with the emotional environment created by the interactions of analyst and patient; it is appropriate if it is indigenous to the unfolding therapeutic process and is not imposed from without. For example, we have reliable knowledge that the function of a transference distortion is to avert anxiety and that the persistent analysis of any facet of a distortion will bring the patient into closer touch with his anxieties. But any attempt to make these anxieties intelligible with an interpretation that runs counter to everything the patient understands about them will reinforce the transference distortion in the long run. An interpretation of this sort never cured anybody, and it may even make it more difficult to study these anxieties in future therapeutic contacts. For better or for worse, moreover, everyone has to work out his own conception of life, and so it seems to be the better part of wisdom to let this happen without any undue pressures and impositions in analytic therapy.

The role of anxiety is centermost in the analysis of transference distortions. Our clinical study requires a set of diagnostic categories that differentiate the many types of personality on the basis of the ways in which anxiety is organized. Diagnostic categories based solely on infantile sexuality, value orientations in later life or some combination of both are actually limited from a therapeutic point of view. They are most useful when spelled out in terms of the organization of anxiety in transference distortions; and of course with the dynamic shiftings of the analytic situation, hard and fast categories are impossible to establish. It has been clinically observed over and over again that any change in the organization of a distortion requires a disorganization of whatever the given happens to be. As an awareness that the customary organization is no longer adequate begins to emerge, anxiety serves as the chief clue that it is breaking down. A psychoanalytic point of view which recognizes the need to reorganize the given will also recognize the need to unravel the various threads of the given; and anxiety is one of our chief guides to the significance of the thread being unravelled.

The study of anxiety in the psychoanalytic situation is an operational one. Regardless of how it is construed, the chief empirical observation we recurrently make about it in the psychoanalytic situation is that it is a function of transference distortions, the detected presence of one leading to the reliable inference of the other. And then the analytic problem is to get at what constitutes the transference distortions, that is, at what the anxiety is all about in that particular instance.

The other analytic approach is to have a definite conception of what ails the patient from the very outset or from the presented history and difficulties. But when followed rigidly, this procedure is fraught with the danger of blinding the analyst and getting him enmeshed in the patient's transference distortions without any firm awareness of what has happened. Because it makes little difference how the analyst is being distorted—so long as one is sure it is a distortion—it is of major importance to find out what has led to the experience of anxiety that has led in turn to the misperception. To get entangled in the contents of the distortion while the patient is undergoing an experience of anxiety of unknown proportions can give rise to transference results in which the analyst becomes distorted in the patient's scheme of things. When this occurs and tends to prevail, the patient will be denied an opportunity to learn about his anxiety with the skilled observer who was supposed to provide him with it; neither the analyst nor the patient is prepared to find out why the transference distortion was necessary in the first place. And strangely enough, in this turn of affairs, the patient's desire to avoid that intolerable experience is actually satisfied while the analyst's concern that he be right about the underlying problem receives the highest priority even though he may be wrong.

Now it is true that we have quite a backlog of information about human troubles and that after a short series of interviews with any particular patient we usually possess enough information to offer some telling hypotheses about his troubles. This may satisfy the symptom-oriented analyst's requirements of having to make the inferences as soon as he has the information and it alleviates the patient's anxiety in the face of his confusion: Someone in authority knows what he is anxious about without his having to tell him; he has found the magical helper who offers him relief without his having to do anything about it. His analyst has been a good doctor who understood the ailment and prescribed the right pills. He has dutifully taken them and reported the alleviation of his anxiety, and both are content—the analyst because he knew the right medicine and the patient because he did not have to do much more than pay for it. And of course the social requirements for being an expert in the field are also satisfied because an apparently desirable result has been accomplished. This is all right if a decision had already been made with the patient that this be the intended goal of treatment. If therapists want to practice that way, there is little to be said about it except that it is not psychoanalysis. The transference distortion of the patient has been satisfied rather than analyzed. But this is not transference analysis in its ideal sense. It may be an ideal that cannot always be achieved in practice with all patients; they are not always motivated by it and the analyst cannot always establish an adequate working base in the mutual endeavor to seek it. And yet the fact that it can and does happen is enough to permit us to outline it as the preferred method of analytic therapy.

Today, twenty years after A. Freud's and Reich's work,[4] the methods of ego therapy and of character analysis are now part of transference analysis. This transition in terminology is by no means accidental. From the middle thirties onward, it has become increasingly clear that the patient's characteristic patterns of disturbance could be studied with striking clinical lucidity in the "me-you" interactions with the analyst and that the most productive way to see them is in this close and magnified transference situation. When skillfully done, it obviates two of the chief difficulties in Freud's hypnotic conception of transference analysis; it limits the projection of the analyst's preconceived metapsychology into the patient's life, and it leaves the reintegration of psychic functioning—the synthetic phase of therapy—to the patient.

Instead of using transference suggestion to overcome resistances so that the problem might emerge into conscious awareness, the analyst now strives to study transference and resistance as soon and as thoroughly as he can. He leaves the resolution of conflict to the patient and uses suggestion as sparingly as possible—only where necessary to alleviate the presenting conflicts. His efforts are exerted chiefly in the direction of transference analysis. It is not the results of reactions, the conflicting situa-

---

[4] *Appendix A,* below, pp. 215–221, is an interpretive placement of their contributions in the perspective of the present study.

tions in which the patient finds himself, that are of primary interest; we focus on his typical modes of reaction, his characteristic styles of integrating interpersonal relations. Of course these resultant conflicts usually constitute the patient's primary motivation for seeking treatment. He usually considers them to be his major analytic problems, and Freud believed that their resolution was the chief task of analytic therapy. From the standpoint of transference analysis, however, the presented difficulties in living are taken as symptoms of the transference repetitions and resistances which will be encountered in the course of the work. The patient's suggestibility is not guided; his resistances are not overcome; his immediate problems are not tackled directly in order to achieve therapeutic goals; our psychoanalytic efforts are not directed toward such ends, since the initial difficulties are viewed as symptomatic of characteristic problems that cut across the typical conflict situations in living. It is the genesis and function of his modes of reaction or patterns of integration that receive our analytic attention. And on the question of suggestibility about which Freud's whole therapy turned, we now look into the patient's surrender of its control and his willingness to allow us to guide it; thus transferences and resistances are intensively studied rather than overcome. The central question we try to pose in each case, then, is why does this person need an analysis of his personality structure rather than what problems in living he would like to have resolved.

Freud noted very early in his work that the therapist's behavior in the analytic situation is of prime importance.[5] Despite the general agreement on this proposition, the full import of his continued failure to analyze positive transference has received tardy recognition. Writings on psychoanalytic technique were extremely sparse after Freud published his theory of transference in 1918, and this may have been rooted in his authoritarian point of view. Experiments were few and far between, and technical innovations were developed very slowly.[6] Those who remained

[5] J. Breuer and S. Freud, *Studies in Hysteria*, New York: 1936, Chapter V.
[6] O. Rank and S. Ferenczi, *The Development of Psychoanalysis*, New York: 1925.

in the mainstream of Freudian psychoanalysis by and large followed the general precepts of the master. The few who dared to attempt independent thinking—like Jung, Adler and Rank in the early years and Fromm, Horney, Sullivan and Thompson more recently—found themselves outside of the pale. If these workers had done nothing more than openly break with Freud's closed system of thinking and therapy, their place in the development of psychoanalysis would have been assured. Differences of opinion were inevitable in such a young and growing science and even Freud's authoritarianism did not obstruct the quest for truth; indeed no single point of view could have been adequate at this early stage in the growth of a science.

Many workers have already commented that analysis of transference as Freud practiced it, tended to infantilize the patient; and Rado has observed that Freud was not as permissive as Breuer was in his earlier cathartic method.[7] Though this may be true, we should not overlook the fact that Freud, despite this personal characteristic, was also caught up in the method he evolved; that is, the patient had to be infantilized in order to achieve the hypnotherapeutic goals which Freud accepted as the essential condition of successful therapy. Why he personally did not surrender these goals would probably take us into the realm of biography. Suffice it to note Rado's observation in this connection, for the validity of the position taken in this study does not require the use of biographical data. Besides, the therapeutic consequences that follow from his authoritarian method may be studied without any excursions into arguments ad hominem.

If we allow for the free interweaving of past, present and future, an entirely new kind of data is made available to us. The patient becomes an entirely different kind of person whose construction of interpersonal problems is usually a valid one in its own terms. If we initially treat him as the adult he is, we do not find him turning to infantile sexual experiences and fantasies. He does not wallow in them because he does not experience

[7] This procedural decision to infantilize the patient derived, of course, from theoretical and therapeutic premises about the relation of change and continuity. Compare, above, p. 23, fn. 4.

them—consciously or unconsciously—as the things that matter most; instead he will follow out the various threads of his problems in the various contexts in which they occur. If the analyst assumes that the patient is interested in exploring his typical personality reactions, he will find the patient ranging through the past, present and future without any preconceived notion of the solely or necessarily sexual etiology of his psychological disturbances. As the analyst canvasses this range of fact, he will find that patterns of interaction can be generalized more and more to encompass wider selections of data; and eventually he will be able to filter out a simplified statement of the patient's difficulties which has been arrived at in common with him. He will not have to force the recall of early memories of sexual or other traumata with the threat that analytic therapy cannot work without it and that if they are not forthcoming the patient is resisting him. He does not have to hold before the patient the absolute necessity of filling the gaps of his infantile and childhood amnesias because he is willing to regard the patient's conception of his troubles as adequate for undertaking the work and for collaborating with him to widen the horizons of his insight.

This approach avoids the following sort of impasse: The patient may not happen to believe that the nub of his problems in living is sexual. In fact, he may even report a rather satisfactory sex life. Now of course he may be resisting what the psychoanalytic authority is telling him to believe. But it may be asserted with equal plausibility that the authority is not able to listen to the patient's report of his experience; the analyst may also be resisting. Why the patient should then be subject to a semi-trance state in order to find what the authority wants or expects him to find in himself is difficult to comprehend; or why the transference is considered negative and hostile and unfavorable to analytic therapy when he persists in his beliefs about his experience has yet to be made intelligible.

This seems to be the heart of the matter. Freud had a conception of why man got into trouble, and the only way he could cure his patients was for them to accept the rightness of his conception. Looking at it in this way explains why Freud allowed the positive transference to unfold without analyzing its distorted qualities until resistance emerged—as if it were not an obstacle to open two-way communication from its very inception—even though it sometimes was too late by then to do much about it. With this positive transference, he acquired a foothold in the patient's experience in order to apply his metapsychological conception of what was wrong. Unfortunately, the patient's wish to understand himself hit a snag in his positive transference, for the analyst, capitalizing on this opportunity, would organize the facts to suit his own metapsychology. And one of those insoluble questions about classical technique may be raised again here: How could the patient's associations be in any sense considered "free" when it was a foregone conclusion that he would eventually learn in the course of the analysis that his associations have to be skillfully guided to the forgotten past and that his recollections have to fit a certain rigid framework?

In effect, however, the positive transference, when it contained distorted dependency needs, was a repetition of the patient's defense against indoctrination, and so he accepted the doctrines of his new adversary on the "battlefield of transference" and vitiated the analyst's power as one human being to speak directly to another. In this transference experience, the patient's reaction to doctrinaire people in the past was duplicated with another person who could not listen to him. The analyst may have been able to sell the patient a bill of goods in this way, but the analysis was bound to fail. For any attempt to get "behind" a defense before there is sufficient common data to call a specific reaction a defense will only evoke more subtle and elusive defensive operations. This procedure can be manipulative, and there will be definite signs of therapeutic success in certain cases. It can produce transference cures in which superficial changes may be observed in overt behavior without tapping their defensive purposes. Such accommodating changes are actually symptoms of transference distortions which require more refined analysis to become accessible. If anything of lasting value is accomplished, it has only been because the analyst unwittingly touched upon the more obscure transference distortions. The alternative to this suggestive process is a careful slow-moving analysis which looks into the defenses without rushing blindly to get "behind" them by anticipating the source of the difficulty. That the patient is defending himself, and that he is defending himself against something specific, have to be studied in collaboration with him.

The fact is that the investigation of any initially presented disturbance in interpersonal relations, past or present, sexual or otherwise, will provide sufficient therapeutic materials for the working out of a general hypothesis about typical patterns of transference and resistance. Curiously enough, where attempts to force the recall of early happenings and fantasies have failed, the operational approach has often succeeded, with increasing insight into a current distortion, in opening up hitherto forgotten gaps in early parent-child relationships. This observation must remain a curiosity in Freud's formulation of transference analysis. If, despite this clinical observation, it is insisted that our efforts be confined to Freud's conception of the procedure, we will find ourselves in a dilemma: to be sure, the patient misunderstands the present in terms of the past, but when he looks into the past he will also misunderstand it in terms of the present. In other words, if the patient distorts his current situation in terms of the past, and then tries to unravel that past through his current distortions, he cannot escape their limitations. It follows that when he undertakes a review of his past he will get caught in a vicious circle; for a past misunderstood in terms of the present cannot throw much light on a present misunderstood in terms of the past. One cannot draw a clear picture of the past until present perceptions are somewhat clarified. This situation cannot be rectified either clinically or logically in Freud's formulation because he required a clarification of the past which is in the first instance simply unobtainable. Now the only way out of this confusing situation is the introduction of other factors into the analysis of transference—the analysis of current transference feelings toward the analyst and future life-goals—to provide a leverage for studying the current dynamic situation so that there may ensue a free-moving interplay between past and future as the patient gains increasing insight into his current distortions.

The most impressive fact we can establish on the basis of this predicament of Freud's technique is that psychological processes are in no sense self-sufficient and self-sustaining irrespective of the other people in the interaction. Psychological methods affect the emergence and selection of the data. As the techniques of inquiry change, the facts inquired into change; in short, psychological observation is participant. There is no absolute and inviolable technique of psychoanalysis which is perfect. Clinical experience has repeatedly shown that if the analyst focusses exclusively on reconstructing the early history, the resistance can operate in current interaction. If he deals exclusively with presently pressing problems, significant genetic factors can be repressed and rationalized to ward off inquiry; but if he has a free-moving approach that is open to the total range of personality development and refuses to be beguiled by content that throws no significant light on function, he can avoid some of the pitfalls that are inescapable in the old free-association-on-the-couch technique.

The last thirty-five years have witnessed a significant reversal in theory and technique. Classical psychoanalysis used to be reasonably sure of its metapsychological explanations of various syndromes and character typology without always being able to do much about them therapeutically. In exchange for this dialectical agility in explanation, we have acquired an increased effectiveness in technique. At the turn of the century, precise differentiation was believed necessary for the development of specific therapeutic techniques to cure specific disease entities. And throughout Freud's case studies, both before and after his self-analysis, we find him persistently trying to isolate the specific cause of the specific psychic ailment. With the increasing recognition of the pervasive similarities among people, we have come to realize that we never deal exclusively with any fixed entities in a dynamically changing picture. It makes little difference that we cannot always make a clear-cut diagnosis between severe hysteria and incipient schizophrenia or between obsessional character with marked schizoid features and pseudo-neurotic schizophrenia; the differential criteria are sometimes very difficult to make out during a diagnostic interview. In any event, we have to deal with the psychological material as it unfolds in analysis. We also know that the analysis of the total personality, genetically and functionally, will disclose diverse syndromes that are diagnostically incompatible with each other but are none the less compresent in the same range of fact about personality organization. This change in perspective has thrown Freud's metapsychological structure into question, and a new perspective in psychoanalytic theorizing has been developing away from static structure in the direction of dynamic process—dynamic process in the therapeutic situation and dynamic process in the development of personality. This study has been more concerned with the field of therapeutic operation than with the general theory of personality development; Sullivan's latest book deals with the latter topic.[8]

We cannot be hampered by any single-factor scheme of metapsychology while we are still trying to build a science. Two idols of early psychoanalysis—the hypnotic conception of transference and the single-factor metapsychology—have been subjected to thoroughgoing scrutiny. In a certain sense, they are closely related to each other. The only way to accept a single-factor metapsychology in order to explain the diversities of human experience is through a trance-like acceptance of what a man like Freud or any other charismatic leader has instructed us to believe. And yet despite the greatness of the man, when his formulations do not accord with the facts of clinical experience, we must choose between our experience or his formulations; and the object of choice is self-evident.

Contemporary psychoanalysts, in surrendering Freud's metapsychology, may have denied themselves the use of an important

[8] H. S. Sullivan, *The Interpersonal Theory of Psychiatry*, New York: 1953, Part II.

tool for getting at anxiety. But they have managed, by taking a pluralistic point of view, to stay closer to the communications of the patient and talk sense to him in terms of them. Many of the sexual metaphors of earlier analytic therapy possessed a certain shock value that sometimes helped to loosen up the patient's defensive system. The free use of interpretations like castration, penis-envy, homosexuality and so on probably had startling effects and produced opening wedges in the patient's defenses against anxiety. But we cannot overlook the other side of the coin: that patients often became panic-stricken when they were told by the expert that they were afraid of losing their penis or wanted a penis or were really homosexual in the absence of confirming facts which could be established by the data already presented. Such pitfalls are avoided with certain patients, the obstacles are increased with others, but the truth must be sought in ways that satisfy the requirements of truth rather than the pragmatic pursuit of flashy results.

The decision on the part of many workers in the field to surrender Freud's sexual metapsychology has been motivated by their perception of what is true in the therapeutic situation. I do not believe that any attempt to psychoanalyze the motivations of workers who seek to improve upon a scientific inheritance will ever succeed in deterring them from seeking warranted improvements. Moreover, those who concern themselves with this sort of psychoanalytic inquiry will never be able to escape the responsibility of analyzing their own motivations for using simplified formulas to analyze the motivations of others in non-analytic settings; and this can only lead to a fruitless preoccupation with matters which cannot be positively verified in the public forum. Besides, it is doubtful that the motivational origins of an idea will ever be definitive when the issue of its systematic and operational validity is at stake.

Freud's attempt to utilize positive transference as an adjunctive tool to overcome resistance was doomed to failure. It had required assertions of authority on the part of the analyst which were not warranted by the clinical facts. We need not belabor the idea that they were incompatible with the freedom engendered by the contemporary scientific and cultural climate of opinion. For habits of scientific technique and communication are in no sense universal in analytic therapy. Even if it were possible for two psychoanalysts to work in exactly the same way, the mechanical self-exertions in this direction would devitalize the interpersonal participation and transform it into an impersonal or depersonalized situation—a rather crude approximation of what a vital interaction between two people can be.

Today, we see rather clearly the concomitant relationship between transference distortions and anxiety—a relationship in which cultural components are the anxiety-producing factors against which the patient is defending himself. There is no need to decide in advance about the nature of these anxiety-producing factors, because in a democratic society where a pluralistic attitude toward life and its values holds sway, many different sources of disturbance may be equally compelling in diverse familial settings. Cultural pluralism thus implies a pluralism in psychoanalytic metapsychology. In practice, this means that we leave the reconstruction of the patient's value-system to the patient and concentrate our analytic efforts on the psychodynamic understanding of his transference distortions. While it is true that every analyst has a system of values in which he believes as a guide to his life, it is also true that he does not have the obligation of imparting all of them to his patients. Even if we analysts were to consider it our obligation to do so, it seems rather futile to work directly with the value-system because it would only make it that much more difficult to get at the basic psychological conflicts the next time a difficulty or discrepancy in value-judgments were to arise. To be sure, when an analyst accepts a patient for treatment, he makes the implicit value-judgment that he has a scientific contribution to make to the understanding of psychological disturbance. But in this pluralistic view of metapsychology, the question of the ethical source of the patient's disturbance is left open. It is not decided in advance that his anxiety concerns any particular sort of experience. The analyst does not have to pre-

judge which area of disturbance he will tackle and help the patient resolve; this is the type of prejudgment that often results in
transference cures. He may allow the patient some real latitude
in his free associations—latitude which many patients are too
frightened to take advantage of—because he has no antecedent
framework into which his patient's problems must fall. And he is
satisfied to seek out characteristic patterns of psychological dys-
function.

Pluralism in metapsychology may eventually lead us to a systematic psychoanalytic science based on the regularity of certain
types of psychological processes, the relationship between transference distortions and anxiety being a case in point. It enables
us to see that differences among the various "schools" of psychoanalysis are essentially differences in the philosophy of personality and life. I suppose that if this point of view were ultimately
pushed to its logical extremes, it would actually mean that every
psychoanalyst constitutes a "school" of psychoanalysis in himself; for a genuine metapsychological pluralism would also imply
freedom of choice for the analyst as well as the patient. But it is
somewhat aberrant to expect the experience of every member of
mankind to fit in every particular into the categories of explanation which Freud had developed to understand himself and his
patients. I have already suggested that the scientific climate of
opinion in which a man lives and works affects his point of view
on the relative value of the various factors in the total therapeutic situation; there is an unconscious patterning of feeling and
thinking which is not easily transgressed. Freud's feat of self-
analysis was prodigious, but he was not able to lift himself out
of his early training in hypnotherapy by his bootstraps; nor was
he able to see beyond the indubitable sexual factors in the etiology of psychoneurosis.[9]

A pluralistic metapsychology alone can avoid the pitfalls of
dogmatism. To apply a single-factor metapsychology to all patients requires forceful indoctrination. It is still impossible to fit

[9] E. Jones, *The Life and Work of Sigmund Freud*, New York: 1953,
Chapter XV, contains biographical information for those interested in the
personal psychology of his scientific formulations.

any single value-system to the vast heterogeneity of life-experiences. The impossibility of this enterprise will become immediately evident to anyone who has ever tried to fit all of his own experience into a single self-consistent system. We have to study life-experience in its actual occurrence; we have to study what makes people anxious without fixed prejudgments in particular cases.[10] We may have our pet theories about the metaphysical and cultural meaning of anxiety which we may not always be able to keep to ourselves during interviews with patients. Yet there is a certain definite sense in which every person has to develop his own personal view of anxiety, not necessarily in any systematic way but certainly in a feeling way. A pluralistic position in metapsychology will allow our patients to develop their own personal metapsychologies that are in accord with their life-experiences. And it will, incidentally, make it possible for psychoanalysts to cooperate more harmoniously as a community of scientists.

[10] For further development of this view, see W. Silverberg, "The Concep of Transference," *Psychoanalytic Quarterly*, XVII (1948), pp. 303–321.

chapter ten

Values in the Therapeutic Situation

EVERY METAPSYCHOLOGY CARRIES WITHIN IT a set of value-affirmations. Explicitly or not, it projects an orientation about the individual and social origins of psychological disturbance, whether they be oedipal problems about sex and authority, the prevailing wish for tenderness and warmth, the socio-cultural organization of life, or any combination of these factors. That patients respond to one scheme of values or another in accordance with the variety of their disturbing experiences is undeniable. The point of view which is applied to the presenting problems of a particular patient often depends on the flexibility with which his analyst can conceive of different matrices of psychological disturbance and the ease with which he can move from one frame of reference to another.

This idea that social values have an important role in psychoanalytic theory and therapy is gaining increasing acceptance. Classical psychoanalysis found itself in the unavoidable dilemma of denying, on the one hand, that the question of values has any place in scientific formulation, while at the same time it could not help but introduce definite social attitudes into its scheme of interpretation. To quote one prominent writer in the Freudian tradition, "a scientific psychology is absolutely free of moral valuations." [1] This position reflected the generally accepted view of nineteenth-century philosophy of science—the neo-Kantian separation of natural science and moral judgment: "facts" were considered to be purely scientific and "values" were practical matters which were anything but scientific. It is doubtful of course that

[1] O. Fenichel, *The Psychoanalytic Theory of Neurosis*, New York: 1945, p. 5.

classical metapsychology was as "value-free" as it purported to be. Freud's dynamic and structural approaches to personality development implied a definite attitude towards man and his place and purpose in the world of the previous century. Yet, because psychoanalytic science was considered to be free of values, the social ideals and affirmations were concealed and defended in a roundabout way.

Any discipline in the study of man which supports this duality of fact and value will find itself excluding scientific intelligence from the active construction of value. This duality defends a theory of value by implication, however. Just as scientific psychology is absolutely free of moral valuation, so the converse may also be true, namely that moral valuations are absolutely free of scientific psychology. But in this latter point of view, since men are in the ineluctable condition of having to do something, the standards of value in accordance with which they carry on their daily affairs are actually accepted on an absolute or uncritical basis. The failure to take account of the possibility that science and value are not so sharply disparate has produced absolutism in metapsychology and authoritarianism in therapy.

Now absolute values in the extreme are imposed and enforced by an outside authority. They are complete in themselves, and prescribe individual acts. There is little room for intelligent discussion: what is to be done is already marked out by an authoritarian fiat, and possibilities which point to other values or even to modifications of the absolute one automatically come to nothing, since the absolute is taken by prior assumption to be final and immutable. The imposed act is its own justification and is simply to be done, so far as any particular person is concerned. Ordinarily, rational analysis depends on the possibility of envisioning connections with other values, but critical thinking is cramped because alternative possibilities are eliminated from values which are intrinsically good in themselves. Where two such values seem to oppose each other, human beings who are not entrusted to weigh logical alternatives must simply carry out a performance which is its own justification. Provisional judgments are indefensible, and any critical sort of theory is impossible; observation is performance, thinking is profession. In this circumstance, the infallible authorities may be consulted for advice which is then to be carried out with a child-like faith in the valuableness of the outcome. Here we find that inscrutable type of situation in which an irresistible force spells out an immovable value. All brands of authoritarianism — political, familial, religious, educational and therapeutic—operate splendidly with this philosophy of value.

The psychological consequences of an authoritarian theory of value are significant for the therapy of adults and children alike. Disturbing situations usually contain possibilities which point to other outcomes, but these latter, though they have equal or superior merit, are left to wallow in the imagination. Since these alternative possibilities cannot be realized in overt behavior without real or imagined danger to the self-system, there occurs a bifurcation of private experience from publicly observed behavior. These covert ideals may someday be attained, but because they cannot be acted upon in the immediate situation, they shrink from overt expression, lose directive traits in social behavior and find a secure haven in private experience. And the stipulated means for the attainment of these unrealizable goals are, by the same token, rendered ineffectual, meaningless and unproductive; for actual step-by-step connections with an imagined goal have been pushed beyond the reach of overt behavior by the authority of the absolute. The idea that things may be valued as goals apart from the accessibility of means to attain them is more than a logical fallacy in practical judgment. For any view of human values which erects an intuited goal as final and unanalyzable and then considers the practical means to its realization as merely incidental will promote submissiveness, hypocrisy or fanaticism.

This celebration of consummate values without regard for the appropriate measures to be taken to attain them may be paralleled with a special type of psychological theorizing. Private experience is, in this theory, divorced from overt behavior and absolute values are placed in "core" experience—only to discover by this assumption that the submissiveness, hypocrisy or fanaticism is merely peripheral: the person is not "really" dishonest, he only acts that way; his use of means only appears to be fanatical, for the ideal is "really" worth any efforts under all factual conditions. But the kind of question evoked by the bifurcation of absolute ends from relative means is equally appropriate with respect to this psychological bifurcation. What can "core" honesty possibly mean if it has no express manifestations in overt relations with other people? How can we assess the validity of an end which never reveals itself but only its peripheral means of realization? And from an empirical point of view, how can this "core" honesty and intuited truth be known and understood if they are not evidenced in interpersonal communication and relatedness? The traditional answer is of course an appeal to introspection as a method of knowing that certain true attitudes or constellations of feeling exist without having to corroborate their existence in the public arena of men. But private introspection is not a technique of scientific investigation; nor is it a method of any interpersonal form of psychotherapy; and all appeals to private experience without recognition of its continuity with public communication and acculturation will at some point actually affirm the authorized ideal which, in the final analysis, simply reflects the express demands of the public authority.

If these theoretical considerations had no practical consequences in analytic therapy, there would be no need to pursue this matter any further. But as we have already seen, Freud's single-factor metapsychology had definite effects on his therapeutic procedure. It leads us to assume that no course of psychoanalytic treatment can avoid dealing with affirmations of value when the patient tries to resolve his conflicts. This assumption will be explored in the following perspective: The psychoanalyst need not make judgments of value for a patient in order to adjust him to the socio-cultural situation in which he is called upon to act. Even if an analyst always could, he need not list beliefs which are normal and compare them with those which are pathogenic, but he is obliged to describe the interpersonal processes accruing to and supporting his patient's convictions, whatever they happen to be. Where clinical formulations about difficulties in living border on matters of social value, it is good procedure to allow the latter free rein. This will permit the expression of more material for clinical observation, and will also enable the patient to realize that concrete attempts to achieve goals are his own prerogative. The acceptance of one mode of social existence rather than another or one cultural aim rather than another is, moreover, not singularly subject to *psycho*analytic description and inference. It is a valuation-judgment about affairs involving information from many spheres of human knowledge other than analytic psychology. Precisely because psychoanalysis has a contribution to make to these judgments of value, it is sought out for clarification of the psychological aspects of difficult human problems. To state this apparent truism would be supererogatory were it not an established canon of classical metapsychology that judgments of value are beyond the pale of science.

The modification of anxiety-inducing conflicts which persist beyond awareness is the valuable thing disturbed people presumably seek in analytic therapy. They seek goals which not only make sense out of their daily activities but also have significance in a wider system of meanings; they seek to secure a satisfactory orientation for the doing of work, the consummation of ends and the enjoyment of living. In the consideration of problems in values, the psychoanalyst centers his attention on the attitudes and feelings expressed towards them. He is especially interested in how the patient approaches their realization and what blocks him in the pursuit of certain goals as compared with others. Thus the goals sought in everyday behavior are not so much at the center of inquiry as the communications about them. For the latter point up the patient's approach to what he desires, strives for and judges worthy in life. Besides, these descriptions of his goals in life and his actual attempts to achieve them often provide important clues about the accompanying interpersonal feelings and attitudes.

At the very outset of analytic therapy, it is usually determined, however provisionally, that certain definite interpersonal difficulties are the reasons for undertaking and undergoing analysis. This provisional and tentative sort of postulation provides a frame of reference in which to assess the future course of the therapeutic work. It is only after the patient has presented his fundamental difficulties that the analyst can make any fruitful contributions about orientations in the seeking of goals. Even though this initially communicated set of goals will not necessarily be maintained throughout as fixed, every attempt at analytic therapy must start with something concrete. In fact, many of these provisionally postulated goals will change with progress in the therapeutic process. These changes in perspective about goals and the manner of attaining them are major concomitants of wider understanding and psychological growth. Indeed successful analysis usually results in a thoroughly overhauled system of values and new attitudes toward their realization; and secure satisfactions acquire a more stable base.

The satisfying qualities of activity are easier to feel than to define. And they are more readily defined in negative terms as activity generally free of irreconcilable conflicts and frustrating predicaments, free of lacks, privations or disruptive integrations; positively, they constitute a feeling-tone of behavior, a sense of significance and well-being. To call satisfaction the supreme goal of human activity arises, of course, from the hedonistic fallacy which confused the goals achieved with the satisfying experience in the achievement of the goal. It would be equally fallacious to reverse the hedonistic position and exclude the sense of satisfaction from the goal which is in fact achieved. The sense of satisfaction may indeed be present throughout every phase of the process as well as the product of activity; it may accompany the quest for means as well as the conquest of ends. But we cannot emphasize this means-ends continuum in behavior to the exclusion of the accruing sense of satisfaction, since both are compresent and mutually compatible phases of experience. When we judge the value of something, the likelihood of its satisfactory quality as an end is most easily guaged, among other things, by its satisfying qualities as a means; and this is implied by conceptualizing means and ends as a continuum. Perhaps the import of this sense of satisfaction would be grasped more clearly if it were used adjectivally to describe its applicability to both sides of the means-ends continuum.

We often observe that certain patients have an insistent need to achieve ends without enjoying the concomitant satisfactions, for some sort of means has been converted into a self-supporting end which is its own ground and justification; that others consistently seem to strive without ever arriving at a terminal point, for they pursue ends which lack any practical means for their realization. Now it is true that certain proposed goals are nonexistent at the time they are considered. It is equally true that some means to achieve them are also non-existent, and even though they are pursued with careful attention to the conditions of their career, they may none the less remain beyond reach. But these are extremes from a logical point of view and not from a psychological one: ends without means resemble means without ends because neither will necessarily terminate in consummatory experiences. If a life is lived in constant search of such values, or if recurrent failure evokes inappropriate feelings, these conditions may provide good—and at times the best—clues to the understanding of why psychoanalysis was undertaken.

William James once used the metaphor of the flights and perchings of a bird to describe the rhythms of experience. In these terms, the quest for values may be said to take place during the "flights," and the achievement of them at the "perchings." Thus the extended activities which are undertaken to enstate a value are consummated in an active closure which marks their actual enstatement. A life that is lived as an endless "flight" or a rigid "perching" in order to achieve particular ends is not exactly worth the interest or the effort, for the good life must feel good as well as be envisioned and proved to be good. It feels good when it is punctuated by integrated terminations at recurrent intervals, and it proves to be good when one gets a feeling of in-

tegrity, worth and freedom from the way in which aims are
realized. The satisfying qualities of these "flights" and "perchings" are to be found in the meaning, ground and direction which
accrue to any organized activity. Without a prudent coordination
of these aspects of experience, human activities become random
movement or blind urgency.

Of course, satisfaction is experienced when a desirable value
is achieved. But since the ground of achievement is not satisfaction but an accurate evaluation of the operant factors and their
projected outcomes, the attempt to attain a value may also be its
own satisfying reward. For the sense of satisfaction is ancillary to
the logical verifiability of the judgment. Although satisfaction is
not itself predominantly judgmental, it is part of the experiential matrix in which judgment occurs. The important fact here is
that the achievement of a judged goal involves a termination of
judgment. The movement is away from deciding how good the
means are, how good the ends are and how to achieve them—
away from trial-and-error testing, careful deliberation and comparative evaluation which are the hallmarks of judgment. The
movement is toward consummatory and quiescent behavior, the
enjoyable feeling accruing to this achievement and enhanced respect for one's capacities—toward the confirmation of one's ability to judge and carry out the implications of a judgment, and
relaxation through the freedom and ease which power to achieve
goals confers on activity. This movement away from judgment
is a movement toward the affective side of experience. There has
been a change in the focus of awareness; its center is no longer
occupied by judgment, for it has given way to consummatory
experience.

In success or failure, a crucial question is whether the value was
a "real" one. It is always relevant to inquire during analysis, once
a goal has been set up as an objective of future behavior, whether
this is what one "really" wants. Now the chief characteristics of
a "real" value are durability and consistency: it retains an enduring claim on one's loyalties throughout a series of diverse
situations. Unlike fantastic goals, it is refractory to psychogenic

analysis. Once appraised and affirmed, it retains its desirability and persists as a goal to be sought; it is adhered to despite variations in tangential characteristics. This raises the interesting metaphysical issue of whether the value is actually the same after some of its characteristics have changed, a question which goes back to the nominalist-realist dispute in medieval philosophy. Fortunately, psychoanalysis does not have to get embroiled in it, for the patient's judgment on whether the goal has remained the same is usually adequate as a basis for continued inquiry. This does not decide the question for the subject matter of ethics, of course. This decision would require an analysis of situations in which ethical inquiry takes place, an analysis which would, on the one hand, set forth the socio-psychological limits of the specific situation and describe the continuity of specific situations on the other. It need not be attempted here since it has little bearing on our immediate purposes.

A consistent and durable value is "real" because it is sought and lived by "stick-to-itively," to use another of James' picturesque expressions. It has run the gauntlet and proved itself to be worthwhile; it has weathered the trial runs to which it has been subjected; it is no longer the kind of value which has yet to be tried —it is affirmed to be true. By contrast, a value is fantastic if it is transient and fleeting; it is "unreal" if its choice, plan or pursuit is recognized as having taken place beyond awareness at some point after a few trials. A "real" value has certain aspects in common with a fantastic one, however. To all appearances, both are selected in the light of intelligent deliberation about their probable consequences and comparative worth. They may both be professed and defended quite staunchly. And tentative efforts may be exerted in their direction in overt performance. Perhaps the basic clues to its "unreality" are the fleeting quality of its occurrence and the unconcern with which it is surrendered. If, on the other hand, failure causes anguish, we must not only reserve our decision about the construction of the value judgment but we must also explore the appropriateness of its emotional concomitants.

A life of enduring "real" values is one in which values are consciously wrought and persistently maintained just because conscious choice has become a sufficient condition of their being sought. Conscious judgment is not the sole conditioning factor of human values, however. They cannot be defined purely in terms of conscious judgment any more than they can be defined in terms of conscious effectivity alone; both conscious and unconscious factors intertwine, as necessary and sufficient factors, in the quest for goals which are not as yet in existence.

All decisions about significant human values are tempered by considerations such as these. And the factor of judgment is a necessary condition because human conduct would become unintelligible if it were interpreted simply in terms of fixed goals whose inherent worth is considered absolute and eternal or in terms of private emotional preferences which are merely expressions of immediate feelings or entrenched prejudice. If a critical theory is to find its ground between these two extremes, it must have room for a kernel of intelligence to account for the placement of values in this range. The varieties of eternal and indestructible standards proposed by philosophy and theology and disposed of by nature and man, the operation of competing moralities in various cultures and in the same culture at different times, and the fact of reasoned achievement in human life—all of these attest vigorously to this fact. Furthermore, even the most cherished "real" values which guide ongoing behavior are, in the last analysis, provisional and modifiable ends-in-view; even the relatively stable and enduring ones are not so rigid or iron-clad that they do not undergo change. If this were not so, the impact of new experience would be rendered trivial. And if they were logically unique to the point of being psychologically self-contained entities, the fact of intelligence would be meaningless.

Moreover, "real" values cannot be defined simply in terms of interpersonal attitudes and feelings. Attitudes are vectors, and they point to specific cultural aims and institutional patterns of behavior through which values are made available. Means to achieve ends are always conditioned by social and cultural factors, and so the means-ends continuum cannot be said to operate in the vacuum of strictly logical or psychological analysis. Ends-in-view thus depend on the availability of means which depend in turn on the life-situation in which the ends are viewed. Ignorance of means or the removal of ends from the reach of everyday life may lead to the acceptance of an impractical way of life, impractical in the sense that nothing in the potentialities of behavior points to its realization.

It is quite obvious that the import of practicality cannot be banished from human experience simply by giving it a bad name and hanging it. Practice means rehearsal, habit, doing, and to call an end impractical simply means that nothing can be done about it, or, conversely, to call it practical implies some concrete deed which answers the question of what is to be done. From this it follows that the deed, over and above the aforementioned factors, confers value on the end. For the end to be a valuable one, it is important that it be accessible in the universe of action, and this in much the same sense that the exertion of one's imaginative powers confers value on it. It also follows that absolute and intrinsic values which are transformed into ends-in-themselves hold very little live significance because no specific attitudes or activities can be brought into operation as means to achieve them. And if such values are none the less maintained, they lead to disturbances in feelings and distort productive aims of conduct.

It need not follow that impractical convictions are to be surrendered solely on the grounds of their impracticality; they may still be deemed valuable even where experience has not hit upon ways or means to achieve them as satisfying goals. To surrender them solely on this ground may simply reflect a loss of faith. Just as the maintenance of aims and convictions for which there are no practical means available can lead to disturbances in living, so a willingness to judge ends solely in terms of accessible means— which I take to be the pejorative sense of what is suggested by the use of "practical"—may also be effective in developing disturbance.

Some of the very great ideals of our Western tradition have been maintained at various points in their history despite the fact that they were considered utopian and unrealizable by the "practical" men of the time. Now such ideals were not products of judgments of value; they have largely been matters of faith. Faith is sustained by the very experience which gives it birth. It emerges out of shared experience and draws upon sources in human culture which are largely beyond conscious deliberation and choice; and only shared experience can produce a vital one which confers a unifying focus and direction on life. But even if faith did not keep unrealized ideals alive, it would still be a psychologically meaningful phenomenon, and would as such deserve a secure place among the other psychological conditions of action. It denotes effective psychological means of forward movement in the domain of being human; and it is one of the denotable conditions which is to some avail in bringing a desirable goal into being. The reliance on faith alone to insure the validity of a goal is an extremely shaky matter, however. The question of affirming one goal or another and considering it desirable cannot be answered solely on the basis of faith alone. The answer to this question depends on the feeling and thinking that one can bring to bear on it from his past experience. To be realizable, the construction of future goals depends upon the substitution of reasoned action for wishful thinking. For faith does not change conditions which confront us; action does, and faith is but one among a multitude of factors affecting decisive action. If faith in visions were confused with actual cultural aims it would make a travesty of value theory and a fruitless pursuit of analytic therapy.

There is another reason why this element of faith has to be placed in its proper perspective in judgments of value. Such decisions are at once personal and interpersonal. Not all attitudes, feelings and thoughts are solely interpersonal in the sense of reflecting the appraisals of others; some need not be referred to interpersonal communications at every point in their process. Occasionally, these decisions for better or worse are made in privacy, even though any one of them is likely to become interpersonal and social as soon as it is acted upon. One may of course discuss them with others in the hope of revising his own opinions or leading them to revise theirs, but making decisions can become a highly personal matter. If this is not always so in fact, it is so as one goal of psychoanalysis, for after all the analytic descriptions and inferences are done, the decisive action is still to be taken in the concrete life-situation without the presence of the analyst. The ethical problem is to resolve the conflict and attain the goal, and describing and explaining the psychological aspects constitute but one phase, however important, of this endeavor.

The purpose of considering values in the therapeutic process is not simply to divide the good from the bad; the purpose is to facilitate decisions for the enhancement of judged goods and the obviation of judged bads. It is necessary to know, for example, which values are major and which are minor, which conflict with or deflect from the realization of an integrated system of values, what implications arise and have to be faced when any goal or set of goals is proposed, what steps of action are required to bring it into being, and whether the available resources are reasonably commensurate with it. The approach to these questions during the early stages of therapy is mainly classificatory; the patient's sentiments, desires, loyalties, strivings, goals and appraisals are noted in order to get a rounded picture of the kind of person being analyzed from the worth he places on his various experiences. The analytic task is chiefly to discern how the person habitually approaches the content and worth of his experience.

While the patient seeks to clarify the known social and interpersonal factors conditioning his judgments of value, the analyst may participate with descriptions and inferences about interpersonal processes. The judged worth of the self is not itself an immediate matter of analytic inquiry, since respect for the personality of the patient implies a respect for the personally and interpersonally judged worth of his experience. It is rather the distortions in the communicated feelings and attitudes that occupy the center of attention, selective or otherwise.

Inferences are made about characteristic traits of feeling and patterns of attitude, and they constitute the immediate domain of the cooperative inquiry which is psychoanalysis. The analyst is not primarily concerned with particular judgments of value which his patients make. He wants to know how they go about making them, whether the environment of people and social norms are deferred to inordinately or whether imaginative resources supply the bulk of immediate prizings, how cultural aims enstated by the group and specific sub-groups are accepted and at what expense, whether likings are deflections of intellectualized patterns of defense, evasions of insight or repressions of feelings, and whether the experiental mood is rigid or flexible, rebellious or depressed, outgoing or in retreat—these are but a few of the subjects of inquiry where interpersonal processes are being presented and described. And he must be prepared to convey his descriptions when the evidence is overwhelming that some significant pattern of attitude and feeling is in operation.

It is obvious that implicit and explicit judgments of value are made by the analyst if only in his conception of mental health. As he participates in the cooperative inquiry, he undoubtedly contributes to decisions on the significance of certain interpersonal processes in relation to others. These judgments are often of a syntaxic kind. Sometimes, however, the phenomena of countertransference, more exactly the analyst's own parataxic tendencies, may enter into his judgment in the therapeutic situation. And this will lead to special complications in the development of the analytic relationship. The absence of value conflicts between analyst and patient can be retrospectively established by the existence of a firmly established working relationship. While they do not have to agree on all values, it seems essential that no serious disagreements arise about the way life is to be lived. Where such disagreements do arise, however, they hamper the therapeutic relationship in many subtle ways. Where the analyst's sympathies and personal distortions begin to operate to the subversion of the patient's, the participant situation will break down or become artificial. The possibilities for empathy—that primary social process by which one persons feels his way into the life of another—diminish. It is most probably an essential condition for empathy to take hold that there be a potential for mutual understanding about important issues which need not be specified apriori.[2] Succinctly stated, empathy is the chief source of hunches, clues and probable hypotheses for selecting and ordering the communicated facts about the patient; it is one source of those leads which constitute the initial phase of all scientific inquiry. But this empathetic attitude does not connote an attitude of blanket agreement, for empathy is not the same as sympathy.

That the analyst be able to feel for the content of another's experience is a necessarily basic, though not sufficient, condition of successful analysis; but his personal sympathies cannot interfere with his selection, organization and appraisal of evidence. If he happens to consider that content to be superficial, disagreeable or of little worth, he will either have to refer the patient to another practitioner or he will find himself trying to impose a new persona on the patient, a persona as artificial, simulated and ineffectual as the disturbed personal organization with which the patient first felt discomfiture. As a result, the patient may appear to be more productive as an analyzed personality, but he will not be a feeling-thinking-acting person in his own right; for this mechanical encrustation—now the analyzed personality—will mask his potentialities for being human as his disturbances did originally.

Where the analyst does not sympathize with the goals of a patient, and such instances occur, psychological analysis of them is not always indicated; if attempted, it would deteriorate into a discussion of why the goal should be sought instead of how to go about achieving it. The presumably therapeutic analysis would become transformed into an attempt to confirm or deny the value of the goal instead of the validity of the inferences about its psychological status and determination. To reduce social goals to their psychological constituents and invalidate their

[2] These issues—the nature of love and friendship, truth and integrity, self-respect and freedom—have already been admirably developed by F. Fromm-Reichmann, *Principles of Intensive Psychotherapy*, Chicago: 1950, in connection with the therapeutic relationship, and by H. Schneider, *Ways of Being*, New York: 1962, in relation to the philosophy of culture and experience.

meaning by way of psychogenetic analysis is an insidious practice. The procedure, perhaps more presumed than practiced, is the psychoanalytic tracing of current attitudes and goals to early childhood experience with a parental figure and then considering them to be countermanded because they are reduced to nothing but involvements with a distorted figure of the past. Curiously enough, though this psychogenetic exploration is often taken to be correct from certain points of view, it does not of itself invalidate the social and personal goals as aims of current behavior. For their validity, urgency and realistic character have yet to be evaluated in their own terms. Unfortunately, many positive feelings towards people and events may easily be disturbed by this genetic and reductive type of analysis.

The evaluation of goals is not a wholly psychological matter, and where disagreement on cultural aims cannot be ironed out, the analytic work will bog down in a dispute over intended social consequences of conduct. These disagreements would exist even if the participants in the analytic inquiry discussed them under non-therapeutic circumstances; they are none the less real for having been introduced into the therapeutic process. If the analyst would like to have his own personal decision in the matter respected, he owes similar respect to the decisions of others. It must be recognized once and for all that the analyst is usually a member of the same society as the patient and that he draws his values from the same culture; they are both subject to its conflicts, prejudices, aims and affirmations. To the degree that these factors are consciously understood, analyst and patient may see through such accoutrements of social life. But understanding does not automatically dissolve them as if through the intervention of magical awareness. In psychoanalysis they are brought to the forefront of awareness to be seen for what they are. Over and above this psychological awareness, one must also proceed to affirm or deny them. After the cultural aims of society are understood from an analytic point of view, they may either be affirmed or denied on the basis of judgments about phenomena, not necessarily or solely of a psychological sort. More often than not, the claim that psychoanalytic science and therapy are "value-free" disguises the operation of uncritically and perhaps unconsciously accepted social presumptions; and such concealment may lead to the dissipation of cultural and institutional categories in a psychic fairy land.

It is doubtful that analytic therapy was ever as "value-free" as Fenichel made it out to be. In Freud's last formulations on therapeutic technique, he plainly stated that suggestion had been rediscovered in the shape of transference. And this can only have meant one thing: that the analyst did take liberties in participating in decision-making in the patient's life, even though he explicitly refused his patient the right to carry out any decisions on his own. If we relinquish the idea that conflicts have to be reproduced solely in the mind, it becomes immediately evident that valid decisions in life can be made and carried out during the course of analysis. So long as the psychological components of the decision are satisfactorily clarified, there is no reason why an important step in life cannot be taken before this process of "reproduction in the mind" which Freud called analysis has terminated. In fact, if the patient is free to act upon his decisions which he arrives at during analysis, he will acquire a new sense of its vital significance. His attempts at psychological analysis are brought into closer touch with his actual life-situation. As a result, they acquire more meaning, and make it more difficult for him to use analysis as an escape from the very things he would like to change. Besides, life does not come to a stop when analysis begins, and analysis, it may be hoped, will continue in earnest after the formal work is done; analysis and actual life-experience may genuinely interpenetrate if the skill of the analyst does not require the erection of artificial barriers between them.

Direct suggestion may of course be used to influence the decisions of the patient but the final act of resolving a conflict is a private one which he may want to do without the intrusion of others; and when he does not, which is more likely to be the case, then is not the objective of analytic therapy to make personal decisions for him, but rather to investigate the conflictual psychological patterns which interfere with his making them. Wherever possible then, the analyst limits his intrusions of precept and guidance into the lives of his patients. Aside from the increased authority accruing to the analyst, this sort of behavior on his part may seem to bring psychoanalytic insight closer to living, but it will actually reflect its withdrawal from the significant emotional problems. A kind of psychoanalytic vacuum may be created which can, of itself, produce new distortions. The patient's sphere of activities may get out of focus and revolve about analytic therapy, instead of having the results of therapy suffuse his daily conduct.

Analytic explanations are best integrated with the everyday problems of the patient as aids in making everyday decisions; but it is the authority of analytic understanding, rather than that of the analyst which enters into the patient's life. The closer analysis gets to living, the further it gets away from historical excavation and metaphorical analogies for their own sake, and the more significant will be its description and explanation of psychological processes for the alleviation of life's difficulties. If considering psychoanalysis involves a decision, if continuing to attend sessions for an extensive period of time involves the repeated affirmation of that original decision, then it is basically in terms of this decision that the analysis proceeds. The analyst concerns himself directly with conflicting attitudes, with tracing their history to the extent to which inference requires, and then turning to the current conflict in a descriptive way. But the actual pursuit of decisions in living is the patient's domain.

No analyst can guarantee the successful outcome of any course of action decided upon by the patient to any greater extent than the patient himself can guarantee it. He may participate in the patient's evaluation of his assets and liabilities, but he participates as an observer, not as a final arbiter on their reliability. He may describe the psychological phenomena which accompany and support appraisals, but he then has to await reports about results and consequences of reappraised behavior. Whether the appraisal turns out to be valid or not depends in part on the preferences and interests which are motives of conduct; in part upon the adequacy of the beliefs about the matters to be encountered in action; in part on the clarity and precision with which the action was mapped out in rehearsal. Its validity cannot be absolutely fixed in advance, but whether it succeeds, fails or yields no decisive results, important clues about motivations may be obtained. The turn in analysis is called by the reported character of the behavior, and the problem then becomes one of exploring why that course of action was taken in the absence of reliable knowledge; for that singular source of corrective knowledge about motivations—behavior—has pronounced its verdict on their character.

Values are established in behavior, and the way to resolve a conflict is to do something about changing the conditions of its occurrence. When a value is projected, the analyst is interested, regardless of whether it is actually enstated, in what prompted the patient to do what he did in such a way as to produce that specific outcome. To be sure, the meaning of values is to be publicly realized and verified in terms of overt behavior. But the distinctive contribution of psychoanalysis to the acquisition of values is the carving out of an intelligible and comfortable status for them in the interpersonal organization of feelings and attitudes. The concern of psychoanalysis, then, is not only with feelings and attitudes about values already established; it is also concerned with conferring determinateness on psychological orientations in life which will provide a desirable base for seeking new ones.

chapter eleven

Psychoanalysis as Science and Art

IT IS DIFFICULT to draw definitive conclusions about the structure of psychoanalytic theory and therapy from a study of this sort. I have tried to present a perspective on the theory of transference analysis which is no longer dependent on hypnotism or the authoritarian picture of the therapeutic relationship for its goals of treatment. Though many clinical changes in analytic method may be derived from this new perspective, it is impossible to conceptualize them in full detail; nor is it desirable, for then we would be saddled with a new dogmatism. These clinical changes have been described at various points in the discussion. It is doubtful, moreover, that any attempt to describe the nuances and contingencies of feeling which arise in the treatment of transference distortions will ever do justice to the live phenomena. The leading principles can be systematized into a coherent perspective, but they hardly take the place of an actual experience of a full-blown transference distortion if one would like to realize how difficult it is to communicate all or even most of its phases in printed words.

This perspective about transference analysis has evolved out of repeated trials and failures with Freud's hypnotic view of the phenomenon. It aims to be free of the authoritarian dogmatism which characterized the analyst-patient relationship when the analyst left positive transference distortions untouched until the patient refused to go along with the analyst's constructions.

There are various metapsychological presuppositions about psychoanalysis as both a science and an art which are involved in the theme of this essay. The most important ones will be spelled out in order to make their meaning more explicit. For this view of the technique of transference analysis will be further clarified by the presentation of some of its basic assumptions.

There is, to my knowledge, no compendium of systematic and formal logic which has been successfully devised and applied to everyday life. And I doubt that a system of deductive principles will ever be worked out for the complete resolution of every specific psychological problem anyone will ever encounter. Such problems are much too intricate and individuated for an exact deductive science. To cover all of their manifold contingencies seems hardly feasible, even if it were theoretically possible. These doubts are fortified by the fact that problem-solving in everyday life manifests no invariant uniformities when viewed either from the side of the problem or from the side of the person intent upon solving it. Even if we could imagine the exact duplication of a problematic set of factors in every detail, the problem-solver would have changed with intervening experience. Thus we are always involved with new and independent variables, and we are constantly confronted with some unpredictable factors in the open future of human existence. However, we do not propose to leave such matters to blind chance or arbitrary fiat on this account. The best available scientific knowledge may still be used to assist us in resolving them. But the fact of time, as a real coordinate of human experience, eliminates any final and formal statement of the principles of a genetic-functional logic. The living dynamism still takes precedence over static logic, and life is stronger than dogma.

This being so, every resolved problem carries its own rationale within it, and external resolutions are necessarily ruled out. To learn how the self-corrective logic of solving human problems works, it is necessary to begin using it in solving a problem. When a problem-solver has thrashed out his problem and resolved it successfully, he becomes more interested in enjoying the attendant satisfactions than in inquiring into his method of inquiry. From a strictly pragmatic point of view, there would be no need to pursue the complexities of this matter any further, for such analyses would only delay the cumulative experience of satisfaction. A satisfied state would only be disrupted by the realization that future experience will bring new matters to the fore; besides, past experience teaches the futility of holding onto problems once they have been resolved. This is the nub of the difficulty so far as the person encountering it is concerned.

But psychoanalysis cannot drop the matter at this point, for its scope includes methodology and technique as well as results. The specific resolution of a problem is taken as an instance of the general pattern of genetic-functional method which does, and legitimately so, become a topic of inquiry itself. Psychoanalysis should pursue this inquiry into the method of problem-solving despite the fact that formal logicians insist upon the divorce of the genesis of an idea from its validation quite vigorously—not so much because the autonomy of our discipline is at stake, but rather because we need to know what has been going on and what is to be done when the patient presents his acute and chronic problems to us for help. Opposed to this aspect of logical formalism stands the unavoidable consideration that psychoanalysts have delved constructively into the historical bases of personality disorders and have cooperated with their patients in effecting favorable reorientations of current functioning. All psychological therapists very quickly find that the formal criteria of deductive procedures cannot be effectively applied to temporally and cumulatively oriented therapeutic procedures, and formal logicians must reckon with the fact that adequate principles of genetic-functional logic which buttress therapeutic inquiry are actually obtainable.

Whether problem-solving takes place under ordinary or therapeutic conditions, it is an art. There is no gainsaying this fact. Like all arts, its procedures and standards in specific situations cannot be entirely legislated for it in advance. On the basis of this notion, we can formulate clinical procedures in the therapeutic situation. Even though psychoanalytic therapy is an art, its objective is to apply specific techniques to specific sets of clinical signs or manifestations of experienced difficulties in each individual case. For clinical techniques which have been forged in the crucible of empirical investigation are designed to deal with specific phases of presented problems. As operational tools to describe and make inferences about disturbed psychological processes, such formulations would obviate many of the problems of formal logic.

When we move from problem-solving as an art—whether it be under ordinary conditions or in therapy—to treating psychoanalysis as a science, we find that we must retain genetic-functional method as the most reliable method of obtaining knowledge for therapeutic purposes. But when we turn from therapeutic art to organized science, we find the following to be true: the observations and definitions of interpersonal phenomena lend themselves to systematic organization which enlarges our understanding of how the patient may become liberated from his distortions and enter upon different modes of experience. And this is the requirement of psychoanalysis as a science. We must assume that people seek its scientific view of why they cannot live their way of life and that they would satisfy their need for other forms of specialized knowledge by consulting other specialists.

The power of a science lies in its ability to discover, establish and confirm relationships among processes and events. In treating the subject matter of psychology as a science, the processes under investigation are found to have relationships which are best understood by distinctively psychological methods, and recourse to the techniques of other subject matters can breed confusion. We may of course introduce factors which operate in other subject matters. But such factors have no privileged status, for we cannot neglect the continuity of processes within the psychological domain.

As in other branches of scientific inquiry, the method and subject matter of psychoanalysis are inextricably intertwined. Distinctive characteristics of the methods of investigating psychological processes are required by the generic traits of the communicational field. Our basic assumption has been that the communicative processes of psychoanalysis possess no differentiating traits which can be described prior to and independently of inquiry, for the results which are obtained are always results of specific investigations. As new and more powerful techniques of exploration are devised, the sphere of understanding and control grows correspondingly, and facts which were previously accepted at face value through habit or custom now become proper materials for further study.

Many of the manifestations of transference distortions have been observed to exhibit certain regularities throughout the life-course of a person, and it is these regularities on which we center our attention. We have been able to ascertain a correlation of processes with unerring accuracy: the concomitant relationship between transference distortions and the aversion to anxiety. This is one kind of established concomitance whose predictability is warranted irrespective of its metapsychological status or how it is used in therapeutic art. Whether distortions become the subject matter for further analytic inquiry or whether they are used as springboards for counter-suggestion, prohibition and authoritative fiat, their function is chiefly to avert anxiety.

From a conceptual point of view, they may quite easily be subsumed under general categories. In Freud's classification, they were divided into positive and negative transference. We have found this to be inadequate. Transference distortions are to be opened up and followed back to a hardly duplicable variety of interpersonal experiences, for the patient as a qualitatively unique person cannot be forgotten. Though the behavioral environment of our patients in their formative years is generally the family, we know today that the emotional environment of each sibling differs despite the general similarity of the ecological environment—so much so that even with identical twins, preferences and goals tend to differ because of the uniquely constructed relationships between parent and child, teacher and pupil, peer and peer and hierarchical position in the group, man and woman and so on. But our aim remains to construct generalized descriptions of transference distortions, even though the varieties of experience which entered into their formation are highly individual and require fine tooth-comb analysis.

The findings derived from such systematic studies in disturbances of personality organization provide some of the important materials for the science of human behavior. Psychoanalysis contributes its share to the understanding of normalities and minor deviations in everyday life by studying the so-called abnormal manifestations. But its contribution to the study of man is more in terms of approach and attitude toward investigation than actually derived results. Its approach to all kinds of human experience reflects a clear awareness of the existence of blinders of a prejudicial sort. It fosters an open-minded attitude of following the lead of a problem without prejudgment. In its refusal to restrict the scope and manner of investigation, it seeks to avoid dictating the experiences man should have by that authoritative bludgeon of "scientific prediction." The analyst must, above all, maintain an attitude of respect for individual difference despite the cultural norms and religio-moral values which he himself may have fallen heir to or adopted. Thus our theory of human behavior needs to be flexible enough to allow the free development of new and hitherto unexpected potentialities, flexible enough to permit the development of new and more suitable techniques of inquiry and treatment; and the techniques must be flexible enough to allow for changes in the disordered process and sensitive enough to detect such changes.

As one of the many techniques available for gaining knowledge about man, psychoanalysis does not exist in a social and scientific vacuum. It is affected by the knowledge accumulated in all fields of science. Continual interplay is thus set in motion between a generalized theory of man and the therapeutic technique of psychoanalysis, a working back and forth between them for mutual benefit.

It is always extremely difficult to state whether metapsychology or clinical experience provides the more powerful impetus to the growth of knowledge. A new discovery in scientific technique may create the need to enlarge our conception of human possibilities; or an enlarged conception of human potentialities and goals may foster the development of a modified analytic technique to bring them within the realm of realization. Freud's description of transference is an instance where empirical discovery preceded the development of a conceptual system and the clinical formulations about its application. And the changes in therapeutic procedures which have been introduced by the neo-Freudians serve as a good illustration of how the conception anteceded the operational procedure.

The specific subject matter of psychoanalytic therapy is defined here as disturbances in interpersonal processes. This definition excludes considerations about ethics, social structure and cultural inheritance from its immediate field of inquiry. Sociology, anthropology, history and philosophy study these matters just as neuroanatomy and physiology study the biological processes of the human organism. The knowledge accumulated in these fields has an indirect and indispensible bearing on the therapeutic interaction as it goes on in contemporary practice. As already indicated, psychoanalysis is interdependent with these other disciplines on a conceptual level as well as in the formulation of therapeutic aims and procedures. Consequently, investigations in any of them would facilitate—but hardly replace—the understanding of personality organization and those characteristic disturbances which comprise the specific subject matter of psychoanalysis. Psychoanalytic therapy is an interpersonal discipline which deals directly with the characteristic difficulties one person experiences integrating himself with another person and participating in this newly integrated situation.

Introspection thus has no place in the method of psychoanalysis. The psychoanalytic situation is first and foremost a communicative interchange between two people, and psychological processes which do not in some way become evident in this interaction are simply unobservable. It is communicative behaviors, the so-called introspective reports, which provide the analyst with his facts of inquiry. Since psychoanalysis, in this approach, studies processes of communication and relatedness which may be observed in factual space and time, introspection can lay little claim to being its established method of inquiry. In the psychoanalytic situation which necessarily involves more than one person, the attempt to observe and interpret one's own feelings and attitudes is bound to be futile. In the first place, the introspected facts cannot be publicly observed because no one is in a competent position to make the same observations and confirm the interpretations. These facts are half-truths which neglect significant aspects of widely practiced scientific procedures. Besides, introspective analysis does not explain why a certain psychological state of affairs exists but only that it is operant in the introspected field and was anteceded by other ones, a psychogenetic regress which may continue with increasing futility until memory fails. But this plethora of details is no clue to the significance of any of them, so far as the analysis of transference distortion goes. And finally, since a transference distortion appears in order to avoid intolerable anxiety, a person introspecting on his own would have a greater stake in ignoring the results of the distortion than in seeing them and letting himself in for anxiety reactions. This, incidentally, is why self-analyses usually fail. In their origin and function, transference distortions are interpersonal, and we have to study them by methods which are interpersonally communicable and verifiable. In view of the confidence and sophistication which have been developed in science over the last three hundred years, we do not expect direct observation alone to verify hypotheses about parataxic distortions.

Of course, a science grows as great insights accrue to and simmer through its structure of knowledge, but its methodology cannot be one which may only be used by rare individuals. Introspective analysis has been carried on successfully by those brilliant students of human experience like Spinoza, Freud and James in psychology, by creative writers like Dostoyevsky, Balzac and Stendhal—in fact, by all original imaginations. These men worked without the active intervention of other people when they took the role and attitude of others toward their own system of actions and attitudes. But after they arrived at great psychological insights, these truths also had to be verified publicly. The point is that all suggestive results of this sort have to be organized and verified by developing a model of interpretation through which observable behavior can be related to insights which are introspectively arrived at. But introspection is unreliable and inef-

990 TRANSFERENCE

fectual in psychoanalysis even when it is the practiced introspection of taking another's perspective toward one's own experience, for this procedure is not the skilled psychological observation and description of interpersonal distortions in their occurrence.

Even if private introspection were accepted as an effective method of psychology, it would automatically disqualify itself from any interpersonal form of psychotherapy. The simple fact is that anyone who has finally sought out the aid of psychoanalytic knowledge and art could not introspect successfully on his own about the distorted aspects of his experience. Obviously, the patient cannot be expected to go the inquiry alone. If he could discern the significant distorted patterns in his system of attitudes and feelings, and if he could decide on the crucial clues to the resolution of his problems, he would hardly be confronting a psychoanalyst with them. As traditionally construed, introspection cannot discover anything useful for an interpersonal form of therapy. The procedures of psychoanalysis involve two people who participate in the relatedness and communication which provide the focal points of the cooperative inquiry. And lest the subject matter of psychoanalysis become amorphous and the art of therapy become the hunting ground of mystics and sooth-sayers, concepts and operations must be communicable, testable and verifiable in all of their significant phases.

Unfortunately, the reliance on communication and relatedness as a point of departure is sometimes regarded as a reductive approach to "mentation." This view is probably a reaction to Watson's rather crude physiological behaviorism. But no account even of Watson's early theories is very illuminating without considering, as their background, the failures of late nineteenth-century introspective and faculty psychologies. Psychoanalysis now seeks to study communicative behavior operationally not because "psychic states" and "mental data" are considered unverifiable in theory but largely because they are unfruitful in practice. The methodological identification of "mind" with interpersonal and social processes of communication has significant value because process is movement and changes in movement are subject to descriptive and inferential analysis. To be sure, "core" dynamics are not always directly identifiable in overt behavior. But once it is recognized that the facts of psychoanalysis can be located in communication and that different "layers" of psychodynamics, so far as communications in therapy go, are actually reflected in different levels of inferential interpretation, the human "mind" may be relinquished as their repository. Interpretation need not be seen as an intuitive way of literally seeing into a person; it can be a technique of getting an increasing number of facts into a wider systematic arrangement by assigning meaning to them at their respective levels of significance.

Communication may be verbal or non-verbal; the significant symbols may be expressive or referential; but relatedness and communication provide the singularly relevant facts under inquiry. Words and gestures are directly observed, and the feelings, attitudes and thoughts which they express or to which they refer are matters of selection, description and inference. The psychoanalyst does not deal directly with and observe the libido, life and death instincts, birth traumas or sex economics. The immediate locus of analytic inquiry is defined and constituted by communicative processes, immediate and referential, for they are the media of interpersonal exchange.

At the same time, however, it would be rather interesting to speculate, in passing, on the probable unreliability and uselessness of some of our most cherished formalities, tonal inflections and nuances of meaning transmitted in gesture, voice and phrasing, and to consider the tremendous knowledge which would be gained about them with more precise physiological instruments. Perhaps the refinement of devices like the electro-encephalograph may some day furnish dependable clues about these intricate facts. But personal feelings and attitudes in the field of communication would still retain their experiential character and be subject to observation and inference so far as anyone else is concerned. The reported measurements of such an instrument would most probably have to be supplemented by psychotherapeutic inferences about transference distortions. In any event, they would have to be checked by the expressed attitude which they presumably measured and reported, if they were to supply additional evidence for characterizing a specific attitude as a parataxic distortion. For there is no compelling reason to believe that distorted fantasies cannot be constructed in the face of neural conditions to the contrary, especially since perceptions about publicly observable matters which are experienced in common with other people are, when needs be, readily distorted.

The structure of psychoanalytic science has been conceived and organized in two essentially different ways: from the standpoint of the genesis and function of the patient's interpersonal processes and from the standpoint of the worth which he places on his experience and mode of relatedness. There are certain types of observation about therapeutic communications which every analyst has made. In Chapter 8, twenty-one observations of transference distortions were noted. They may be made by workers with metapsychological points of view which are basically different from the one which is taken here. But these observations stand no matter the metapsychological point of view. And though the operational definition of transference which I have offered may not suit all workers, it is the most precise I have been able to construct. Needless to say, it is open to revision if found cumbersome or imprecise. But the major criteria to be used in evaluating it are its accuracy in description and value in application.

Turning our attention to the analyst's own distortions, we find that these observations and definition of transference can easily be converted into the observations and definition of countertransference. The difference between transference and countertransference as observed and defined is solely the person about whom the observations and definitions revolve. What happens to these processes in the therapeutic situation presents a much more radical difference between them. Once the observations of countertransference are made, they may be introduced into the treatment situation in order to add to the patient's data on his transference distortions, and for this purpose alone. For even if the patient were not caught up in a transference distortion, he has no obligation to help the analyst clarify his countertransference problems. The analyst's clarity about his countertransference may enable him to get at important clues about the patient's contribution to the interaction, assuming he has some reliable understanding of what it is about others that evokes this kind of reaction from him. But so far as the structure of the processes is concerned, transference and countertransference, it is maintained, are similar, the chief difference being whether it is the patient or the analyst who experiences the parataxic distortion.

Cohen has set forth a series of observations of countertransference which parallel most of the observations of transference noted in this study.[1] Their interchangeability can easily be demonstrated by inspection:

(1) The patient expresses an unreasoning dislike of the analyst.

" (1) The analyst has an unreasoning dislike for the patient."

(2) The patient describes the analyst as unreal, mechanical or depersonalized. When the analyst makes a comment or asks a question designed to gather more information, the patient tends to ignore its point while seeming to respond to it.

" (2) The analyst cannot identify with the patient, who seems unreal or mechanical. When the patient reports that he is upset, the analyst feels no emotional response."

(3) The patient becomes overinvolved with some personal trait of the analyst that has little if any bearing on his experience or skill—or even on the patient's ability to work with him.

" (3) The analyst becomes overemotional in regard to the patient's troubles."

(4) The patient expresses excessive liking for the analyst, feels he is the best or only possible analyst for him, and claims that no one else in the world could assume and successfully carry out the therapeutic task.

" (4) The analyst likes the patient excessively, feels that he is his best patient."

[1] M. B. Cohen, "Countertransference and Anxiety," *Psychiatry*, XV (1952), p. 241.

(5) The patient dreads the hours with the analyst and is persistently uncomfortable during them.

" (5) The analyst dreads the hours with a particular patient or is uncomfortable during them."

(6) The patient is preoccupied with the analyst to an unusual degree in the intervals between sessions and may find himself imagining remarks, questions or situations involving the analyst. The analyst may appear in the patient's dreams as himself.

" (6) The analyst is preoccupied with the patient to an unusual degree in intervals between hours and may find himself fantasying questions or remarks to be made to the patient. . . . (16) The analyst appears in the patient's dreams as himself, or the patient appears in the analyst's dream (Gitelson)."

(7) The patient finds it difficult to focus on any aspect of his problems. He is vague about them and discusses them as if he were consulting the analyst about his case as one professional colleague to another.

" (7) The analyst finds it difficult to pay attention to the patient. He goes to sleep during hours, becomes very drowsy, or is preoccupied with personal affairs."

(8) The patient is habitually late for appointments or shows other disturbances about time arrangements, such as running over the end of the hour or saying that he does not want to leave. Any disturbance about any aspect of the arrangements, once entered upon and mutually agreed upon, fall into this category.

" (8) The analyst is habitually late with a particular patient or shows other disturbance in the time arrangement, such as running over the end of the hour."

(9) The patient continually argues, seeks love, remains uninvolved or indifferent about important problems in his life—in fact, continually does any one sort of thing in an automatic way.

" (9) The analyst gets into arguments with the patient."

(10) The patient becomes defensive with the analyst and exhibits extreme vulnerability to the analyst's observations, inferences or interpretations.

"(10) The analyst becomes defensive with the patient or exhibits unusual vulnerability to the patient's criticisms."

(11) The patient consistently misunderstands or persistently
requires further clarification of the analyst's interpretations.
When he never agrees with them, this transference process can be
tested simply by repeating to the patient an observation of his
own which he had made earlier in the hour—and he will usually
disagree with that too.

"(11) The patient seems to consistently misunderstand the
analyst's interpretations or never agrees with them. This is, of
course, quite often correctly interpreted as resistance on the part
of the patient, but it may also be the result of countertransference distortion on the part of the analyst such that his interpretations are actually wrong."

(12) The patient seeks to elicit a particular emotional response from the analyst—for instance, by provocative remarks,
double-edged questions or dramatic statements.

"(12) The analyst tries to elicit affect from the patient—for
instance, by provocative or dramatic statements."

(13) The patient becomes overconcerned with the confidentiality of his work with the analyst.

"(13) The analyst is overconcerned about the confidentiality
of his work with the patient (Fromm-Reichmann, personal communication)."

(14) The patient beseechingly or angrily looks for sympathy
regarding some sort of maltreatment, real or imagined, at the
hand of some authority figure.

"(14) The analyst is angrily sympathetic with the patient regarding his maltreatment, real or imagined, at the hands of some
authority figure."

The other seven observations of transference noted in Chapter 8
could just as easily be converted into instances of countertransference. These twenty-one observations are, I am sure, but a partial
list of the multitude which have been made.

This transformation can also be effected with the operational
definitions of transference and countertransference. The defini-

tion of the former: *When in the patient-analyst relationship, the patient's anxiety is aroused and interferes with continued collaborative endeavor on the problem at hand, the alteration of the patient's behavior, verbal or otherwise, is a transference distortion, the emergence of parataxic communication in the therapeutic situation.* And the definition of the latter: *"When in the patient-analyst relationship, anxiety is aroused in the analyst with the effect that communication between the two is interfered with by some alteration in the analyst's behavior (verbal or otherwise), then countertransference is present."* [2]

By listing these observations and definitions together, we see one striking fact from a systematic point of view: transference and countertransference are bipolar or reciprocal phenomena. An axiom may, therefore, be set forth which will intergrate these sets of observations and definitions into a coherent system, and it may be called the axiom of mutual or reciprocal relations. With respect to transference and countertransference, this Axiom enables us to structure and organize the many observations and the two operational definitions. It organizes and simplifies them, since the axiom is implied not only by the derived definitions but also by the first-hand observations.

This is an axiom about the genesis and function of processes observed rather than about their metapsychologically viewed content. It is one in a series of axioms which may have to be constructed in order to integrate our observational and inferential knowledge. Processes like resistance and security operations, for example, require similar logical and systematic treatment. If this axiom of Bipolar or Reciprocal Relations will embrace operational definitions of the latter processes, it will prove satisfactory; if not, a new one will have to be constructed, and then we will see whether a higher order of postulation will systematize these axioms. There are, then, different orders of postulation in psychoanalytic science. Tentatively, we classify them as follows: first order of factual observation, second order of operational definition, third order of axiomatic postulation, and possibly fourth order of postulational integration.*

[2] Reference footnote 1, p. 235.

* See, below, *Addendum* (1964), p. 199.

Psychoanalysts ordinarily restrict themselves to the first order of observation and description and the second order of operational definition with their patients. But these have not proved sufficient to organize our knowledge into a structured science; the one picks up directly observed and described facts in the therapeutic situation for the purposes of understanding and perhaps influencing a recurrent type of disturbance, and the other organizes these facts into a body of knowledge about the specific disturbance; the first order is literally first and the second order is second in the temporal order of knowledge. These two phases of inference are always subject to modification as new evidence is observed and interpreted. The systematization of second order inferences into a body of knowledge to which first order inferences may be referred is a logical matter which requires more than the utilization of first order descriptive data in the therapeutic situation; it requires our proceeding to higher orders of postulation. This system of psychoanalytic definitions may provide a rationale to explain why specific sorts of therapeutic efforts lead to personality changes, but the first order description of therapeutic evidence alone can provide an understanding of the important question of how such efforts produce reconstruction and change.

From the second order of postulation onward, this attempt to systematize empirical observations and definitions may be open to the criticism of divorcing the study of interpersonal processes from their socio-cultural contents and products. However, there are a number of comments which may clarify the position taken in this essay and perhaps anticipate this line of criticism. First of all, there is really no such thing as psychoanalytic sociology. To avoid any misunderstanding, I would like to state categorically that the study of interpersonal processes cannot be divorced from the study of social organization. There is a definite need for intervening scientific constructs which workers trained in both psychoanalysis and sociology seem best qualified to satisfy. In so far as current methods of investigation permit us to study them, the categories of one are not interchangeable with those of the other. The bridge between them cannot be built if it is based

upon an uncritical merger which overlooks crucial and generic
differences in their subject matters and their special techniques
of investigation.

Secondly, the express aim of the above attempt at theory construction has been to exemplify the structure and organization of
psychoanalytic knowledge. Psychoanalysis is first and foremost a
study of interpersonal processes. So far as the scientific side of
the matter is concerned, the aims, products and evaluations of
these interpersonal processes are to be supplied by other disciplines. No self-respecting psychoanalytic scientist will make judgments about matters of physics, biology, physiology, sociology,
economics, education or ethics whenever he really has no technical competence in these fields. A systematic theory of man does,
of course, point to a multi-discipline approach which may some
day provide information at each point of convergence of these
various sciences and at the appropriate order of postulation; the
content of the process and its goal in action will determine the
kinds of information required and the science which possess it.
In the absence of any such systematically codified science of man
which can provide the answers, psychoanalysts, by and large, rely
on common sense—let us hope it is sense of a not too common
variety. The slow rate at which such a systematic science is developing suggests that analysis will be relying on a commonsense
view of things for quite some time to come; hence the need for
unassuming self-critical appraisals of the value-system by which
each individual analyst lives and works.

And, finally, it is the belief of this writer that the aims and
goals of the patient's interpersonal processes are ultimately his
own domain of final decision, the analyst's value-system and commonsense view of things to be contrary notwithstanding. In fact,
did a codified science of man exist from which the analyst could
deduce valid judgments about specific events in his patient's life,
the final decision would still rest with the patient. This view of
the matter is based largely on three considerations—the value
judgment that must be made that each person has the last word
on the interpretation of his past experience and the determina-

tion of its future course; the empirical fact that within certain limitations man can choose between alternatives with which life presents him and that this choice in life cannot in any total sense, be controlled by any other person—witness psychosis and suicide; and, finally, even though this structure of psychoanalytic knowledge requires highly general axioms twice removed from concrete therapeutic observations about interpersonal processes, its method of inquiry throughout is inductive as well as deductive—at once public and self-corrective, its operational definitions being open to revision with the appearance of new observations.

In forswearing dogmatisms and authoritarianisms of all sorts, scientific method has its burden of proof in a special perspective in the philosophy of science, one which is naturalistic, humanistic, democratic and self-corrective, one which celebrates human powers of growth and forward movement in social and personal affairs. It is perhaps best to close on this note, that this view of scientific knowledge in psychoanalysis, as in any other human domain of inquiry seeking to lay bare the intelligibility of nature to the mind of man, presupposes a system of values which not all investigators consciously share but to which they are bound every time they undertake any scientific sort of investigation in any field of human endeavor.

[*Addendum* (1964): At this fourth order of postulational integration, the notion of the shared experience or the experiential field of therapy is suggested in B. Wolstein, *Countertransference,* New York: 1959, and is more fully elaborated in B. Wolstein, *Freedom to Experience,* New York: 1964. Transference and countertransference, in this conceptual scheme, are operational terms of the second order, while their coincidence as reciprocal or mutual transactions is of the third order—which means, in effect, that while distorted transference is indefinable apart from countertransference and distorted countertransference is indefinable apart from transference, neither participant is capable of engaging in mutuality before both resolve their reciprocating distortions. This radical relativity of transference and countertransference, however, requires a postulate at the fourth order like the shared experience or the experiential field of therapy to account for their coincidence as reactive functions of each other in the first order of observation and description.]

Appendix A

From Id Therapy to a Therapy of the Total Personality

To THE DETRIMENT of theory and as a complication in practice, the immediate aspect of distorted transference has yet to receive the attention it deserves. In so far as it characterizes the patient's personality in action, it resembles any other of his recurrent patterns; and its distinctive mark for psychoanalytic inquiry, of course, is that its troublesome consequences also operate beyond his awareness and control. The failure to deal with this resemblance would be difficult to understand were it not for the historical accident that psychoanalysis developed at the outskirts of general psychology and, therefore, was rather hard pressed to carve out a unique field of inquiry that in no obvious way replicated any already in existence. Though this sort of historical view may reasonably account for this omission, it still falls far short of correcting the resultant and widely current production of unanchored psychoanalytic theories. For what is more important in the analysis of distorted transference, as in that of any psychological pattern that has to be reconstructed, is that it has to be experienced openly and directly, its meanings have to be worked out over and over again, and its anxieties have to be resolved simply and squarely in the patient's relationship with his analyst. Only as it comes increasingly into focal attention and under conscious control does it also become subject to organized change, but its qualities of plasticity and stability are no different in kind from those of any other integrative pattern, emerging under similar conditions of origin and functioning under similar conditions of relatedness and communication. As it moves in awareness from the unconscious fringe to the focal center, it begins to resemble any other psychological pattern so that, eventually, it can be reconstructed in the same ways. Such a view of transference is at least implicit in all psychoanalytic inquiry, else all efforts at making its distorted aspects conscious would be misguided and misspent. A detailed exploration of this view will be undertaken in order to describe the gradual movement of psychoanalysis from a therapy of the id to a therapy of the total personality.

Even though Freud did not always welcome observations, procedures and theories that differed or diverged from the singular direction of his growing system, he was clearly the last to treat it as a catechism. Simply to paraphrase his contributions, therefore, as though they could provide for every conceivable situation of psychoanalytic therapy, now is hardly a sensible course to take. Nor would it be productive to rearrange or rephrase them in a dialectical way for the sole purpose of retaining a vestigial linkage with his thinking. Such approaches do his conceptual system the grave injustice, curiously enough, of distorting it through a retrospective misreading of his theoretical and practical intentions from the standpoint of later experience and knowledge that were not his, and they also lead later inquirers into the dangerous trap of appearing to understand what still is beyond the grasp of established procedures. Indeed, to consult and follow his views without a pattern of reconstructive analysis that is open to new clinical observation and inference, even would make a travesty of his original discoveries and be a betrayal of his scientific integrity. It is with the aim of perserving the essential kernel of Freud's contributions to clinical inquiry that the classical system is repeatedly subjected to careful review—no more, no less than those of ego psychologists, character analysts and interpersonal therapists who have followed him—for in this spirit of free inquiry are the hope and the challenge of any future psychoanalytic therapy.

In Chapter XXVIII of his *Introductory Lectures,* Freud declared that the procedure of psychoanalytic therapy is based essentially on suggestion, and he then set forth the distinction between the direct use of suggestion in hypnosis and the indirect form of suggestion to be used in psychoanalysis.[1] This was very much a required and illuminating distinction because it drew a clear and abiding line between the two therapies; yet it also implied that both used a common method of suggestion, only in different ways. To describe psychoanalytic suggestion as being indirect does not suffice, however, for it may be used indirectly and also be distorted. Hence, the importance of supplementing the classical distinction of direct from indirect suggestion with that of genuine from distorted suggestion in order to define it in psychoanalytic therapy, at least ideally, as being both indirect and genuine. That is to say, the analyst does not aim his suggestion directly at the active conflicts with which his patient is struggling; rather, he aims it at the unconscious psychic operations that serve to maintain them, with the proviso that his indirect suggestion requires the support of clinical observation quite apart from his patient's reactive and irrational dependencies in the therapeutic transaction. The practical aspects of this proviso cannot be over-emphasized, since the vestiges of hypnotic suggestion that Freud had used in his prepsychoanalytic procedures, continued to insinuate themselves into his later therapeutic conceptions, in spite of the clearcut line that he drew between direct hypnotic suggestion and indirect psychoanalytic suggestion; and late into the thirties, even, are these vestiges discernible in his writings. When he first had set recall of lost memories and conquest of resistances as the central goals of psychoanalytic therapy, he actually was still pursuing the original goals of hypnotherapy—which, to his way of thinking, remained the same throughout his lifelong study of the psychoneuroses.

To the historians of psychoanalysis, it probably will always remain an enigma that Freud finally failed to free his therapeutic conceptions from hypnosis and from its procedural goals. And the enigma only becomes increasingly obscured by the fact that he could demonstrate far more daring in the metapsychological realms of speculation. Abundantly evident in his historical rec-

---

[1] S. Freud, *A General Introduction to Psychoanalysis*, Garden City: 1943, p. 390.

ord, however, is the swift expansion of his interests to other fields
after the 1915–1917 *Introductory Lectures* which contain his fullest statement of his therapeutic conceptions. There are, for example, the many important works of the twenties and thirties
such as *Civilization and its Discontents, The Ego and the Id,
Group Psychology and the Analysis of the Ego, The Problem of
Anxiety* and the *New Lectures* that gave ample testimony to an
expanding metapsychological outlook, but he unfortunately did
not turn it back into a corresponding expansion of his therapeutic outlook. Thus, even though he had laid out the foundations of his ego psychology, outlined the workings of the repetition compulsion beyond the pleasure principle, emancipated his
theory of anxiety from complete dependence on libidinal pressures, and applied his psychoanalytic philosophy to social and
political psychology—all of which signified rather sharp breaks
with his previous positions in metapsychology—he did not alter
his therapeutic framework systematically for the inclusion of
broader aspects of the patient's total personality. Nor did he
modify the procedural goals that he had originally inherited from
hypnosis and later continued to pursue in his basic model of
psychoanalytic therapy, so as to have allowed, encouraged and
even required attempts in such a direction. Instead, to the very
end, he remained loyal to the supremacy of historico-genetic
procedures.

Historically, all of Freud's modifications, enlargements and revisions of psychoanalytic procedure gave rise, in short, to a theory
of therapy that he had developed as far as he was going to take
it by around the end of 1917. This means, in effect, that all
analysts who begin where he left off, no matter what they believe
about metapsychology, have to start with that particular theory
of therapy which, as we have seen, itself consisted in modifications, enlargements and revisions of late nineteenth-century approaches in hypotherapy. Now, some analysts prefer to work with
the clinical conceptions as Freud left them in his *Introductory
Lectures;* others continue to modify them strictly in accordance
with his contributions to metapsychology during the twenties and

thirties and in accordance with the terminology of his original
frame of reference, as well; and still others now work with the
psychological field of inquiry he so inventively had pioneered,
using his basic tools of observation and inference to construct
new therapeutic perspectives that can be derived through the
analysis of transference and resistance, but an analysis that no
longer is chained to his preferred slant in metapsychology. To
those who still like to consider the science and art of psychoanalysis a finished piece of intellectual architecture, laid out and
built up to suit unchanging blueprint specifications, the subsequent history of psychoanalytic therapy has been a series of rude
shocks, sometimes stormy, sometimes misguided and always lurk-
ing with heresy. Perhaps Freud was a bit more sanguine about
such eventualities, for he had intimated his expectation that the
metapsychological map of the human domain was hardly ex-
hausted by his own: he saw the structure of psychoanalytic
inquiry defined as a matter of procedural facts—namely, those of
transference and resistance—even though it arrived at other results.[2] The results he was referring to, here, are metapsychologies
or philosophies of human nature or culture, while the distinctive
mark of genuine psychoanalytic inquiry, he held, was the intensive investigation of transference and resistance in the therapeutic
field. When he wrote this in 1914, he had yet to work out his
theory of the total personality—but it probably would have made
little difference if he had, since the therapeutic core of psychoanalysis may be realized independently of it, and other results
in metapsychology are compatible with the special character of
psychoanalytic inquiry. From the historical circumstance that he
devoted the last two decades of his life largely to the formulations of metapsychology, it obviously does not follow that his
clinical formulations were finished and done with, once and for
all. Though he did not reformulate his definitions of transference and resistance since his 1915–1917 *Introductory Lectures*,
others already have done so in various details and in various

2 S. Freud, "On the History of the Psychoanalytic Movement," *Collected
Papers*, Volume I, London: 1950, p. 298.

perspectives, and they continue to make these definitions the central core of psychoanalytic inquiry, as a distinctive procedure of psychotherapy.

It therefore is constricting and even misleading to assume that the psychoanalytic character of a therapeutic procedure is at all a metapsychological matter; it is far more constructive for the future of this field to take both the clinical facts the analyst, as analyst, singles out for attention and the procedures he uses to work with them, as the structure of psychoanalytic inquiry. Aside from the social theory of personality, for example, to which Sullivan hitched his notion of "transference-distortion," [3] the main value of his new terminology of prototaxic, parataxic and syntaxic communications was to reinforce Freud's realization that the practice of psychoanalytic therapy could result in metapsychologies other than his own. The particular historical relevance of Sullivan's notion of parataxic distortion, then, was to assert the metapsychological neutrality of the transference phenomenon, and emancipate its observation from interpretive entanglements with the libido theory—which, for systematic purposes, suggests that the notion of "transference-distortion" be used in the therapeutic field and that the notion of parataxic distortion be used more generally in the study of communication at large. This neutral perspective on metapsychology, moreover, reopens the question of values, sentiments, preferences and prejudices to the pluralism and diversity that each individual patient brings to his

[3] H. S. Sullivan, *Conceptions of Modern Psychiatry*, Washington: 1947, p. 4. Among the post-Freudians, Sullivan worked out the most systematic application of this new perspective to the therapeutic field. His notion of parataxic distortion freed the analysis of transference from dependence on the libido theory. But he did not explicitly distinguish it altogether from metapsychology; rather, he posited an inborn "power motive" (p. 6)—which, if not handled with care, easily could become the theoretical agency for but another biological transcript of a culture's values in the psyche and, therefore, but another metapsychology of power. Yet, because he no more used the "power motive" than he did the notions of need and security as mediating terms in his therapeutic conceptions, he belongs to the psychological wing of psychoanalysis.

therapeutic experience: it is no longer a foreclosed issue, at least, that his experience automatically will fall under the interpretive categories of any single metapsychology.

A. Freud's ego psychology, Reich's character analysis and Sullivan's interpersonal therapy all continued through the late thirties and into the forties to transform the structure of psychoanalytic inquiry—a gradual transformation with certain aspects of which Freud, incidentally, seemed to be in genuine sympathy even though he did not contribute substantially to the application of these therapeutic frames of reference. Sullivan's work may be placed in this context, it is proposed, because once Freud had dissociated his theory of the ego's structure from the metapsychology of instincts, the difference between the ego and the self-system was far more a question of interpretive schemes than one of clinical observations. In that period, the trend of psychoanalytic thought was beginning to move in the general direction of the patient's integrative patterns of relatedness and communication, a movement that reached a natural and fruitful terminus in the early fifties when the analyst's personal involvements in the therapeutic field began to be treated more openly, and the therapeutic field itself to be viewed in the round as a total field of total personalities. This gradual change came about in response to an increasing awareness of the fuller implications of participant inquiry—namely, that just as both participants instituted and transformed the experiential conditions of psychoanalytic therapy, so they also shared a participative responsibility for its successful resolution.

In view of the varied and radical changes that the structure of psychoanalytic inquiry has undergone during the last fifty years, the problem that analysts now face and have to deal with seriously, is whether drastic reformulations of entire frames of reference are always needed to meet recurrent breaks of therapeutic practice from the molds set by previous analytic formulations and, when attempted, whether tremendous expenditures of time and energy to construct such reformulations can be justified by the meager results. It may be too early in the history of psychoanalysis to decide which is preferable, if only because the last word in philosophical psychology has yet to be written. May it not prove more fruitful and more economical to maintain a continuity of basic procedural terminology instead, while continuing at the same time to reconstruct its meaning and to refine its application? The view of this study is an attempt in this latter direction, with transference and resistance taken as the central terms and conditions of psychoanalytic inquiry and without any pejorative judgment made of the varieties of metapsychology in which such inquiry is carried out, as long as the therapeutic experience is explored as fully in depth and in breadth as its participants can go.

In the early days of psychoanalysis, the tendency was to be rigid about sexual metapsychology, stretching its application to cover the whole range of human nature and culture and illustrating it with an equally thoroughgoing application to the analysis of each patient's experience of transference. As one result, however, since transference was regarded as being very intimately intertwined with infantile sexuality, its analysis was dominated by the search in early trauma for historical origins of disturbance and distortion. But with the rise of character analysis in the late twenties, that of ego psychology in the early thirties and that of interpersonal therapy in the early forties, the study of the patient's transference was expanded to include patterns and directions of everyday life, bringing them into therapeutic range in terms of the armor-plating of his character structure, the defense mechanisms of his ego or the security operations of his self-system. This very significant modification of therapeutic procedure was highlighted by a rather amusing contribution to the metaphorical traditions of psychoanalysis: Freud's "egg" now was spiced with Reich's "onion." But this change in metaphor also symbolized a serious change in the organization of actual inquiry: it no longer sufficed merely to crack the ego's shell, and get a direct line to the memories of early childhood; it also was now necessary to examine the integrative patterns of relatedness layer by layer, starting from the peripheral present in which the patient was involved and step by step, moving around and backward to the infantile center of his experience. In constructing theories of psychoanalytic procedure, the utility of such intuitive metaphors may be questioned, but the value of these symbolized changes of actual procedure is beyond question. The new views of the ego which Freud had been developing since the early twenties, were reconstructed in various ways by A. Freud, Reich and Sullivan and were then applied for the first time to the systematic treatment of the patient's experience. There now were two parts into which they divided the analysis of transference or "transference-distortion"—the "shell" and the "egg" itself or the self-system and its envelope, the personality—separate and distinct yet in some sense still rooted in an instinct or need theory.

By the early thirties, then, transference was divided into two parts and both were interpreted to have their origins in the past. In A. Freud's terms, there were "a libidinal or aggressive element, which belongs to the id, and a defense mechanism, which we must attribute to the ego,"[4] each requiring its own appropriate procedures. This statement of the issue marked a significant breakthrough, though at the time, it fell short of dealing explicitly with transferences of the superego in their own terms. In any case, whatever view is taken of classical metapsychology, it still cannot be openly adopted and be rigorously applied so as to compartmentalize clinical observations in a simple one to one correspondence with the categories of the id, the ego and the supergo. Though, in classical thought, the phenomenon of transference carried a fairly stable genetic denotation, it has no such label attached to it when and as it appears in the therapeutic field. Historico-genetic analysis, moreover, is rarely observed to resolve a central and compelling distortion because it fails to encompass a patient's integrative psychological movement into his future. A distorted transference emerges in the therapeutic field, therefore, in ways that are much the same as those of any other pattern of

4 A. Freud, *The Ego and the Mechanisms of Defense,* New York: 1946, p. 21. By permission of International Universities Press, Inc.

the total personality, and it does so because it is the same as any other such pattern. Nothing of therapeutic significance can be gained, then, from treating it any differently—not, certainly, in the treatment of character disorders and schizoid personalities where, in the nature of the case, the problems of genesis no longer can be resolved in genetic terms and where problems of function, if thoroughly clarified, may yet be resolved in future fields of experience. Such a resolution also relieves the patient of repeatedly having to return to that past for clarification since, in fact, a significant psychological pattern of the forgotten past is neither past nor forgotten but, instead, continues to unfold in the present beyond conscious awareness. What the classical analyst designated as transference, actually, was nothing more than a firm and ongoing pattern of belief which a patient had developed in early childhood about the integrative range of his operant self and which he later enacted in the therapeutic field as a pattern of his now distorted self.

With the introduction of character analysis or ego therapy, the reconstructive value of a direct and thoroughgoing response to later patterns of development, in addition to those that had their origin in the distant past, was finally established by means of appropriate procedures. This conception was not carried to its logical conclusion, however—a fact that did not become clearly understood until the fifties when, as a result of further accumulation of therapeutic experience, the impact of the analyst's personality gradually came to be acknowledged as a significant factor in his patient's efforts at self-reconstruction.[5] Nor, as already noted, did the bifurcation of transference into "a libidinal or

[5] For sample writings about this theme in various perspectives of metapsychology, see P. Heimann, "On Countertransference," *International Journal of Psychoanalysis*, XXXI (1950), pp. 81–84; M. Little, "Countertransference and the Patient's Response to It," *International Journal of Psychoanalysis*, XXXII (1951), pp. 320–340; C. Thompson *et al.*, "Symposium on Countertransference," *Samiksa*, VI (1952), pp. 205–228; M. Cohen, "Countertransference and Anxiety," *Psychiatry*, XV (1952), pp. 231–243; L. Tower, "Countertransference," *Journal of the American Psychoanalytic Association*, IV (1956), pp. 224–255; and B. Wolstein, *Countertransference*, New York: 1959.

aggressive element, which belongs to the id, and a defense mechanism, which we must attribute to the ego," suit this later stage of therapeutic observation, since patterns of transference have aspects of both as well as of the superego. Yet, if this duality of transferences were consistently used in actual practice, it would tend to distort the patient's communications about himself in the therapeutic field, systematically separating into two "parts" what he actually experiences and reports as a disturbing unity. Under psychoanalytic conditions of inquiry, the id's impulses are not observed to exist apart from the ego's mechanisms that organize them for both repression and expression—wherefore, the attempt to analyze them in abstracto as transferences of the id may only freeze the therapeutic procedure into an artificial mold whose significance for the live problems of experience has yet to be established. Instead of an artificial separation which introvertedly directs the focus of awareness into the vortex of a disturbance that itself is not artificial, the quest for psychological leverage to reconstruct established patterns of relatedness, and plan still other ones, has proved to be far more productive; for id transference and ego transference and even superego transference, together, encompass origins and dynamics, current functions and future purposes. By their repeated communication a patient intends, among other things, to bridge the experiential gap between himself and his analyst, while the cool detached response of straight mechanical analysis would tend to deaden the felt urgency of the problem, yet without loosening the constrictive knots in which it tied up spontaneous behavior, since its obsolescence as an immediate therapeutic concern need have no significant correlation with the obsolescence of its behavioral effects.

Ordinarily, this distinction between id transference and ego transference, whatever its theoretic value, has little direct bearing on any pattern in respect to a patient's experience and report of its disturbing qualities. The analyst therefore tries to respond to it as a unitary communication with one of his own, thereby avoiding the sort of standardized cliche that would distract his patient's attention from what ails him. Such a unitary response also may encourage the patient to pursue even further his exploration of that and of other repressed patterns of impulse and thought so that these, too, may finally enter awareness here and now and in the foreground of the therapeutic field. Through the openness of the exchange and in the security of the therapeutic relationship, a patient may get the courage to penetrate further into the more painful sectors of his experience, now and then, here and there, to discover the felt structure of his experience as well as he can. It would be an unfortunate waste—the work having come to this point—not to pursue further the private terms of his individuating self. Even the most cursory acquaintance with psychoanalytic therapy would reveal that these experiences of selfhood cannot be made to order in the therapeutic field to fit a certain metapsychological mold. When they do appear even in rudimentary form, it is not always as important then to know why and how they emerge as it is to acknowledge and respond to their emergence in vivo—and it is far more important to learn what else there is to be communicated before attempting to switch over into reflective inquiry. Their history and organization indeed do have therapeutic significance, and when such factors are brought into the focus of awareness in terms of their still current effects that are capable of communication, the analyst is ineluctably bound to respond in some way—directly, indirectly or silently—to the unfolding of these self-characterizations, whether or not he would call his patient's immediate attention to their known past structure or to their current behavioral implications. After such experiences are undergone and worked through current fields of psychoanalytic inquiry, they also confirm the fact that characteristic patterns of a patient's past may continue effectively to operate in his current life, and that intervening experience has not proved sufficiently constructive toward their modification. As such private notions of selfhood begin to take conscious form and to have a structural impact on the total therapeutic field, including the individuating traits of the analyst's personality, the essentially therapeutic pulse of psychoanalysis may be said to come alive.

At such points, the analyst's response is generally crucial, not only affecting the immediate outcome of the particular transaction but also setting future guidelines for the collaborative inquiry. In effect, he contributes to the structuring of their ongoing relationship, and influences the expectations his patient may continue to have of him. Moving onto this new ground and toward him to reintegrate the relationship from his side, the patient assembles these various psychoanalytic responses into an unconscious apperceptive screen of communication so as to grasp these ordinarily unintegrated aspects of himself, and sustain their relatedness. This rather significant development usually takes place during the early phases of the therapeutic work: it is variously referred to as "testing the limits," a phrase that suggests the competitive aspects of the culture in which both analyst and patient live, as "denying dependency" when the authoritarian-submissive axis is singled out for emphasis, or as the "honeymoon" to emphasize the sexual or libidinal aspects of the therapeutic field—in each instance depending on the metapsychological perspective in which the therapy is interpreted to take place. No matter the metapsychological perspective, however, the empirical fact is that the patient has to discover for himself whether he can get his analyst to know him—which, in effect, requires him to get to know his analyst—and whether he also can communicate his problems in ways that are meaningful to his analyst and to himself; he did enter psychoanalytic therapy, after all, because he wanted to get some help with them.

What light does this view throw on an already complicated therapeutic situation? Its special relevance is the metapsychologically neutral perspective that it sets forth about a shared therapeutic effort into which both participants, in the course of constructing a field of relatedness and communication, project their cherished values, sentiments, preferences and prejudices. The assumptions of any particular psychoanalytic metapsychology in that field are more a function of any particular analyst's beliefs about the nature of human nature than they are a function of anything supposedly inherent in the nature of psychoanalytic inquiry; but his own metapsychology will remain relatively constant, of course, as he moves from one patient to another, or from one phase of the work to another with a single patient. Glover has summed up this point, stressing the operational factors that now are recognized as present in every psychoanalytic inquiry: there is no aspect of psychological functioning that cannot serve the purposes of psychological defense and hence give rise during psychoanalytic inquiry to manifestations of resistance.[6] Though he did not assert the independence of this proposition from any single metapsychology—in fact he affirmed the classical instinct theory as his metapsychology, and used the libido theory in his therapy—it contains the seeds of a genuinely psychological approach to psychoanalysis, and may be adopted without adherence to any metapsychology in particular.[7] Under the conditions psy-

---

[6] E. Glover, *The Technique of Psychoanalysis.* New York: 1955, p. 57.

[7] It remains one of the more obscure riddles about the development of classical psychoanalysis that one eye could continue to ignore what was plain to the other. Though the metapsychological eye has been fully conversant with the death instinct for about forty years, the therapeutic eye has been glued almost entirely to the libido theory: the wish for sexual intimacy with the analyst is widely recognized by classical-minded writers, while they do not give equal attention to the wish to do him violence, or to destroy him. Freud, of course, never actually assimilated the two into a single focus in his therapeutic conceptions—which may be why it still is possible for some biological Freudians to practice out of the libido theory, at the same time affirming a dualistic metapsychology. In fact, his formulations of the psychoanalytic process in the 1915–1917 *Introductory Lectures* were based largely on the libido theory—which would imply a single instinct theory for therapeutic procedure, and he never returned to those *Lectures* to reformulate his therapeutic conceptions, and fit them to his later metapsychological dualism of eros and thanatos. Hence, the biological Freudian who, when he took aggressive factors into account, may have thought that he was following in the footsteps of his master, was in fact overlooking the meaning of death within his own perspective, as an instinctual force in the therapeutic field. The psychological Freudian, on the other hand, did not have the problem of applying this theory in his practice because he did not use either of Freud's instinct theories—the first dualism of sexual and ego instincts, or the second, a dualism of life and death—to interpret aggression and violence—instead interpreting them as reactions to fear, frustration and inhibition.

choanalytic observation, then, any psychological process may become a defense against the actual awareness of any other; and no process is immune from this eventuality. In short, with or without libido theory or instinctual dualism, this procedural judgment holds for any psychological process as encountered, observed and described in the course of psychoanalytic therapy. It may be invoked, moreover, to explain the well known interminability of analysis, since the defensive context of any process always remains open to change and to further inquiry, while a decision to terminate the formal psychoanalytic work represents a developed capacity to deal with this interminable defensiveness, as posited in the structure of personality. Even though there is no aspect of its function that cannot serve the purposes of psychological defense, it is a structure, nonetheless, of which the defensiveness is an ongoing function. Otherwise, psychoanalysis would be bound to an interminable chain of psychological processes, each moving from one therapeutic context to another but none stabilizing a point of reference about which to undertake comparative analyses of the varieties of defense that are instituted at various times and places, with various types of people, in various ways. Nor could their concomitant disturbances at origin or in consequence be evaluated in terms of the strenuous efforts that would be involved in their analyses—that is, there would be no way to decide the comparative worth of undertaking psychoanalysis as over against attempting to do something else.

But from the further fact that such defenses give rise during analysis to manifestations of resistance, it also may be inferred that the notion of resistance has to be generalized. If the first part of Glover's assertion about the ubiquity of defense is brought to bear on therapeutic constructs and checked through the structural point of view, then a view corresponding to the unity of id transference and ego transference will have to be formulated about the observations of resistance. To illustrate this more concretely: it has become an established practice, since the work of A. Freud and Reich, to distinguish resistances due to distorted transference of the ego's defenses from those arising out of repetitive transference of the id's impulses; that is, the classical concept of transference was set off into two types expressly to accommodate two types of psychic process. Such a distinction may be supported, of course, by a metapsychological system, and Freud's theory of personality does in fact require it. Yet this, in itself, does not suffice to justify the multiplication of constructs in actual psychoanalytic procedure, unless commitments to the biological side of his metapsychology are strong enough to displace the desire for conceptual simplicity in the ordering of psychoanalytic observations. For while it is true, when the ego's defense mechanisms are differentiated from aggressive and libidinal elements of the id, that it is also necessary to differentiate resistances due to the former from those that are due to the latter, this theory of therapy still leaves a vacuum in the study of both—which is represented, in classical terms, by the notion of the superego. This vacuum, it may be speculated, was a direct result of the classical analyst's decision, as a procedural rule, to replace his patient's knowledge of himself with his own knowledge of him.[8] Instead, that is, of treating a patient's value judgments as but another source of psychoanalytic material, the analyst took it as his therapeutic objective to join forces with a patient's superego in the analysis of the id's impulses and of the ego's defenses —his expressed purpose being to "serve the patient in various functions as an authority and a substitute for his parents, as a teacher and educator."[9]

On the other hand, it is also clear in the classical formulation that resistances due to transferences of the ego are both defensive and repetitive, just as resistances due to transferences of the id are both repetitive and defensive. Inspected more closely, therefore, and without apriori commitments in metapsychology, this distinction breaks down: it would attempt to differentiate in theory what it cannot differentiate in practice—a differentiation, in this case, that makes little actual difference—and, rigorously applied, it could needlessly hamper steady observation during

8 S. Freud, *An Outline of Psychoanalysis*, New York: 1949, p. 72.
9 Reference footnote 8, p. 77.

clinical inquiry. No matter how the metapsychological status of resistances is construed, then, it is practically self-evident that they are stubbornly in the service of defensive repetition, and even become refractory to any sort of theoretical interpretation. Nor is it infrequently observed, the analyst's preferences in metapsychology aside, that the obduracy of resistance is enforced as a therapeutic reality by an unconscious interlocking of transference and countertransference. Thus, even if, following the classical structuralization of the ego and the id, a practicing analyst found it necessary to posit the facts of transference and resistance as separate and unrelated facts, he would then have to disregard his preferred metapsychology in order to deal directly with the anxiety that is encapsulated in this converged resistance of transference and countertransference. In any event, this bifurcation of resistances according to their metapsychological source into radically different types is required by Freud's instinctual mythology —which, it is clear, compels the analyst to cut a patient's communications to fit biological patterns of interpretation.

Any approach to psychoanalytic therapy that slights or ignores the obdurate qualities of a patient's resistive defenses, of course, is out of touch with therapeutic realities.[10] Yet, this is not the central point at issue; the question, rather, concerns the procedural possibility of setting off these two types of resistance from each other while the patient is undergoing a felt compulsion to

[10] Whether this defensiveness is an enduring fact of contemporary culture —dominated, as it is, by the "industrial-military" complex—or whether it would also be a normal phase of development in a relatively noncompetitive culture, remains an open issue in the context of this discussion. It is not necessary to get involved, here, with the details of this issue, though it would be in a study of personality theory. No matter how the sociocultural aspects are decided, when defensiveness arises in the therapeutic field, it has to be treated as naturalistically as any other psychological process in the therapeutic field. And what an individual patient can actually do in the analysis of his defensiveness, at present, remains an individual matter that is to be decided empirically: it is never deduced from a philosophy of cultural criticism; it can only be determined according to each therapeutic field of transference and countertransference.

resist. What, in other words, is the therapeutic value of the analyst's using preestablished systematics as the substance of his response? All that need happen in the patient's experience, for him to be able to follow out the systematic line of his analyst's interpretation, is a dynamic shift from the mode of felt immediacy to that of reflective analysis. But neither logically nor psychologically does this entail a corresponding shift in his defensive system from resistance to productive inquiry. If, indeed, he were in true resistance, he might easily interpret his analyst's interpretation as but the analyst's defense against his own sense of futility and desperation about the resolution of his patient's resistance, by which manifestation of counterresistance he would deflect the emotional outpouring of a resistive process rather than admit defeat and helplessness in the face of its obduracy, or with which he might even distort it so as to counter the possible intimations of therapeutic failure and tragedy that, in dealing with disturbances in living, sometimes are just unavoidable—any of these the patient may come to believe, because his analyst may want to protect his own view of himself as a competent practitioner of his art. It is therefore a patient's blindspot about his analyst's concern, for example, that is the substance of his resistance—and not related to the ego's defense mechanisms or to distorted impulses arising out of a chaotic and timeless id, except by a wide stretch of the theoretic imagination.

The notions, then, that the ego's defenses be treated apart from the aggressive or sexual elements of the id, that in any analysis of the total personality the one can be separated for study from the other, that transference of ego defenses can somehow operate independently of transference of id impulses and, conversely, that the id processes in continuity with those of the ego (even with those of the superego, which the original formulation of ego therapy omits from its procedure) are absent from the patient's very first contacts with his analyst—all these are artificial and have failed to be demonstrated. No less artificial is a psychoanalytic approach that would begin with the opposite aim of ignoring the obdurate qualities of a patient's resistances; it is no less wooden, myopic and out of touch with therapeutic realities. In such fields of inquiry as these, the therapeutic work may turn into an intellectual game in which the metapsychological determination of a resistance becomes far more important than the resolution of its compelling anxiety, essentially a game of chess in which it is more important to know the moves of the various pieces than it is to win the game.

Clearly, the analyst's naming of genetic sources of a resistance, or his choosing its name from between ego transference and id transference, has very little perceptible effect on its immediate function—except, perhaps, to contribute to the formation of another layering of resistance. A transferred resistance is a unitary pattern that the patient brings into focus when and as he experiences a denotable wave of anxiety in the therapeutic field. It is, however, a total pattern, and though established psychoanalytic metapsychologies would treat it as being made up of certain constituents rather than others, it is a pattern whose origins and functions may best be understood as a unit of relatedness that is called to the fore under determinate therapeutic conditions, some of which have been supplied by the analyst in and through his participant communication. The goal of its analysis is not served by first breaking it up into many small pieces and then translating these into many other things the patient does not recognize himself to have meant, especially if he cannot correlate his experience with the metapsychological terms in which the analyst dissected it to his awareness. Even though these many components may eventually come to the foreground of his awareness after that foreground has been carefully explored along unconscious lines, if they are not already present, there is no a-priori reason to assume or to impute their presence until the patient begins to become aware of his own metapsychology. He usually has some notion of why he lives through the total pattern in the way that he does—a notion with which it is better therapy to start, since it is his own, than it is to put it into the categories of his analyst's so far unrelated metapsychology. In taking this course, the analyst has contributed toward an increased probability of mitigating and of resolving the transferred resistance. By working directly with its observable functions, as distinct from its hypothecated constituents he helps to make it clear that the resistance has it origins within the context of his patient's experience, no matter how its constitution is metapsychologically interpreted. If he were to become entangled with interpretations of those constituent elements before his patient had the opportunity to work them through to a reading of his own, the analyst would effectively provide his patient with still new points about which resistance could come into play, meanwhile losing track of the original resistive experience whose constitution, he would claim, he was only trying to examine. But if he withheld his metapsychology for its duration, interventions of this sort may even prove unnecessary because the patient will then be able to make his own interpretations, and set forth his own beliefs about the integrative focus of his psychological self, within the context of a personally derived metapsychology. The genuine problem the patient has to face, therefore, is to understand the how, the what and perhaps the why of his resistance as a function of his distorted self. In his therapeutic work, the classical analyst must have encountered the special effects—the derivative resistances, that is—of his metapsychological interventions, no matter how conscious or mirrored were his procedural intentions. If he considered this the sole and necessary procedure, of course he had to undertake it, accepting these added resistances as unavoidable consequences; but what he considered necessary, another analyst may consider a merely arbitrary pursuit of traditional metapsychology raised to the power of unquestioned belief.

The classical practice of separating a patient's repetitive and defensive projections into two types of resistance, in addition, underestimates the value of sustaining the immediate therapeutic context in which they are being communicated. This limitation is further compounded by the radical shift it brings about in the patient's mode of awareness—from that of immediacy to that of reflection—and before he can get a rounded sense of their immediate operations, his analyst's urgings in the direction of historico-genetic inquiry have foreclosed the immediacies of the issue in that therapeutic field. To develop this further, let us briefly reconsider the notion of transference in its traditional sense of affects displaced from the past, as distinct from the later dual theory of transference that included transference of the ego's defenses, as well.[11] Between the time of the original occurrence of those affects in childhood and the time of their presumed recurrence in the therapeutic field, however, a complicated structural development has intervened—which, in classical theory, was described as the ego and the superego. Since every sort of resistance is communicated in and through the screen of this structure, and since any one may be observed throughout the analysis to occur in continuity with any other, they can be described as cooperant and unitary events, and treated as functions of each other—the whole process as a unitary one of transference-resistance.[12]

The fact that psychological processes can acquire a defensive aspect in the therapeutic field, was recognized very early in the history of psychoanalysis, and Freud had devoted a paper to this problem in 1894.[13] But his observation, unfortunately, only

[11] This theme has already been closely examined in B. Wolstein, *Freedom to Experience*, New York: 1964, Chapter 2. It may be noted, here, that when resistance is defined as a function of transference, neither of these terms is now used as they were used in the frameworks of id therapy and ego therapy.

[12] Though this view is implicit in A. Freud's work, she did not make it explicit. After sighting the operational similarity of defense and resistance— "since it is the aim of the analytic method to enable ideational representatives of repressed instincts to enter consciousness . . . the ego's defensive operations against such representatives automatically assume the character of active resistance to analysis" (*The Ego and the Mechanisms of Defense*, New York: 1946, p. 32)—she was prevented from simplifying the definition of this major term of psychoanalytic inquiry—by, perhaps, adherence to the classical metapsychology of personality. Nor, by the way, did Fenichel later simplify it in his codification of classical psychoanalysis (*The Psychoanalytic Theory of Neurosis*, New York: 1945, p. 24 and pp. 571–572). By permission of International Universities Press, Inc.

[13] S. Freud, "The Defense Neuro-Psychoses," *Collected Papers*, Volume I, London: 1950, pp. 59–75.

presaged increasing reliance of his psychoanalytic procedure on
the military metaphor and on its power-oriented climate of
relatedness. Even a cursory review of his later case histories would
confirm the impression that his patients were exposed to an intensive and forceful process of reeducation, on the assumption
that they could not be cured until they suited their experience
to the measure of classical metapsychology.[14] Unconscious processes were treated as though psychoanalytic understanding of
them depended upon the acceptance of his jealously guarded
metapsychology in fine detail, yet because adoption of a firm and
unremitting therapeutic attitude was also a norm of military procedure, this itself may have reinforced a patient's defensiveness
that, in turn, hardened a sense of certainty into an authoritarian
stance that, in turn, reinforced the defensiveness that, in turn,
reinforced the authoritarianism, and so on into a spiraling coil of
therapeutic communications until analyst and patient had moved
so far into struggle with each other that they eventually lost sight
of the intial point of their meeting; instead, they were now embroiled on the "battlefield" of therapy over the analyst's application of his instinctual metapsychology.

It was, no doubt, out of an abiding respect for the defensive
potentialities of his patients that Freud adopted the authoritarian stance. Yet, in such a therapeutic atmosphere, the military metaphor of "battle" and "defense" still needed a third term
—unexpressed but operant, nonetheless—to round out this description of psychoanalytic procedure, and that term could only be
"attack." Thus, after the classical analyst recognized that any
psychological process, in the service of "defense," could obscure
the universal instinctual theory whose application was very clear

---

[14] See any of Freud's case histories in his *Collected Papers*, Volume III,
London: 1950, especially his "Fragment of an Analysis of a Case of Hysteria,"
pp. 13–146, for a first hand impression of this pervasive quality. For further
comments on Freud's study of Dora, see, above, pp. 52–58. And for the types
of therapeutic transaction that may be attributed to the aggressive and
authoritarian analyst, see B. Wolstein, *Countertransference*, New York: 1959,
Chapter 4.

to him, he resolved to mobilize a therapeutic "attack" in response to his unrelieved fear of succumbing to a patient's boundless resources for "defense." Why, in brief, was the classical psychoanalytic procedure formulated in military terms with transference as its "battlefield," to follow a single strategy of "overcoming resistances to recall," and gain a special sort of victory, "recover lost memories?" The answer may be given in terms of culture and in terms of procedure, but it may also be given in those of psychology: the classical analyst seemed to be far more concerned about structure than he was about function, constancy than change, stability and security than plasticity and risk—more, in short, about the past than about the present—when the psychoanalytic experience itself is actually the creation of what will later become a new past, and not just a duplicate creation of the prepsychoanalytic past—which, alone, explains why it enlarges the range of future possibilities.[15] No other approach was open, however, to a single minded analyst who believed in the universal application of a single factor metapsychology to the structure of therapeutic inquiry, to the theory of personality and its development: he appeared to move inexorably along a single track through the diverse and plural existences along the way, constantly reinterpreting their meaning to fit them into his universal theory. And today, as well, the analyst who believes he has a private lien on the universal truth, still cannot emancipate his therapeutic approach from authoritarianism.

15 For further discussion of this last point and of the relation of possibilities and probabilities in psychoanalytic inquiry, see B. Wolstein, *Freedom to Experience*, New York: 1964, Chapter 5.

Appendix B
Structure of Psychoanalytic Therapy

IT IS CURIOUS that the therapeutic significance of immediate experience has escaped serious attention until very recently in the history of psychoanalysis, especially since direct access to it is far more characteristic of clinical inquiry. This gross neglect probably resulted from the steady focus of classical psychoanalytic procedure on genetic roots of psychological disorder, rather than on current functions or expected consequences.[1] Without regard, in principle, for the patient's immediate context of action, the classical analyst shied away from the unconscious present in which distorted transference actually takes shape and, perhaps as a consequence, from the conditions of countertransference that help to shape it in the process of being related and communicated. Any therapy of the id, however, has to bypass the life situation in which the patient goes about his daily business and is compelled to act; it even approaches the point of interpreting such activities pejoratively as "acting out," on the assumption that unintegrated and unsocialized forces of the id are somehow observable

[1] For a recent restatement of the classical Freudian position, see K. Menninger, *Theory of Psychoanalytic Technique*, New York: 1958. It continues to leave unanswered central questions about the role of time in therapeutic experience—the critique of historico-genetic procedure by I. Macalpine, "The Development of the Transference," *Psychoanalytic Quarterly*, XIX (1950), 501–539; the progressive aspects of transference in H. Nunberg, "Transference and Reality," *International Journal of Psychoanalysis*, XXXII (1951), pp. 1–9; the irreversibility of temporal movement by E. Levenson, "Changing Time Concepts in Psychoanalysis," *American Journal of Psychotherapy*, XII (1958), pp. 64–78; the emphasis on the dynamic present in D. Lagache, "Le Problème du Transfert," *Revue Française de Psychoanalyse*, XVI (1952), pp. 5–115; or the role of the future in R. Schonbar, "Transference as a Bridge to the Future," *American Journal of Psychotherapy*, XVII (1963), pp. 309–324. For an alternate view of psychoanalytic process as moving from past, through present, into future, see Chapter VI, above, pp. 83–99.

in a pure state, or can be studied apart from all other psychic processes of the total personality: it gives rise to the old line about the patient who has to stop living until he finishes his analysis.

That the procedures of psychoanalytic inquiry are essentially clinical, and distinct from the mathematico-experimental ones of the laboratory, by now is probably and practically beyond dispute. First and foremost, the procedures of psychoanalysis are experiential, while their subject matter is made up of processes that are both direct and immediate and reflective and discursive; hence, quantitative analysis of clinical observations fails to encompass immediate and dynamic aspects of shared therapeutic experience as these are peculiarly available in psychoanalytic inquiry. The relevance to psychoanalytic therapy of standard postulates of behavioral inquiry is negligible, if only with respect to inquiries into immediate qualities of transference and resistance and also with respect to actual changes these inquiries effect in the structure of awareness. Not that the mathematico-experimental procedures of behavioral science are so highly specialized; rather, that the analyst knows this formal discipline to be the swiftest way to lose touch with his patient, and disrupt the special nature of his own type of inquiry—first turning the field of therapy into a patterned charade to fit its operations and results to certain metapsychological requirements and then turning both participants into depersonalized units in order to avoid the direct impact of face to face experience. Thus, even though the analyst appreciates how other subject matters ordinarily gain recognition as behavioral science, he still has to work with the special traits of his own, and follow its leads in the formulation of procedure. Otherwise, he ceases to do what psychoanalysis does best—inquire at first hand into human experience as lived and suffered—for his alone among the sciences of man dips into the stream of immediate experience without being able to control the initial conditions of every therapeutic effort and without having the freedom to experiment for its own sake where viable human values are involved.

There is still no substitute, in any case, for a direct clinical experience of treating a particular patient, in respect to the type of empirical operations by which clinical inferences can be made and supported, or the type of systematic hypotheses that are most useful for enlarging the scope of clinical observation. Here, the best generalization about psychoanalytic inquiry is that every transaction of a particular analyst with a particular patient is basically concrete and, from the standpoint of its immediate aspects, sui generis. As long as the immediate aspects of therapeutic experience are studied dynamically and structurally, the validity of absolute metapsychological principles is difficult to demonstrate or to corroborate. The continuing search for absolute or quantifiable entities has doubtful value, moreover, in a psychoanalytic procedure whose goal it is to comprehend a shared field of experience. To adopt these methodological limitations does not involve the surrender of other conditions of empirical inquiry; it merely underlines the inferential status of principles derived by observation and description. The therapeutic relativity of transference and countertransference suffices to provide a factual basis for the testing of theoretical assumptions about the psychoanalytic process. It follows, then, that unchanging generalities about the etiology of psychological disturbance and metaphysical absolutes about the human condition are both open to serious question, and this point will be considered below.

Analyzable factors of the psyche, unlike those of physis, are still incapable of being treated axiomatically and exhaustively. This is recognized by any practicing analyst who does not feel inferior about the comparative status of his science or, on account of this, feel pressured to distort his subject matter to suit the requirements of physical science. A psychological table comparable to the one Mendeleef constructed for the elements of chemistry, for example, is not currently attainable. Under laboratory conditions, of course, it is no great feat to combine or to separate the discrete elements of hydrogen and oxygen, but isolable factors of personality under observation in psychoanalytic therapy are not subjected so easily to analysis, control and prediction.[2] Perhaps because it now is almost standard practice to attempt a duplicate of major therapeutic observations in the format of laboratory experimentation, the genuine complexities that arise in actual psychoanalytic inquiry are frequently lost sight of. At present, at any rate, it has to be taken simply as brute fact that precision about psychic process differs in kind from what is available in physical science or, even if this difference were somehow overcome, that exact quantification has limited value for psychological growth. In the therapeutic field, moreover, to the extent

[2] In progress, today, is a rather curious dispute between those who view the therapist as a "behavior control machine" and those who believe the essential fact about a therapist to be that he is a "spontaneous person" (see L. Krasner, "Behavior Control and Social Responsibility," *American Psychologist*, XVII (1962), pp. 199–204). But both are wrong for, oddly enough, the same reason: the analyst may be just what he is and need be nothing else, if he would not become any more confusing to his patient than he already is by virtue of his patient's distorted potentialities; yet, because he is a therapist, he has to have a trained ability—best, perhaps, when it is unself-consciously used—to carry through a psychological investigation of personality from the standpoint of the patient's reconstructing his distorted self. Though the "behavior control machine" would probably be an impossible person, and though the "spontaneous person" might do just as well bartending, such private reactions are quite aside from the main point—namely, that the whole dispute between the two centers about a faulty premise they have in common: no patient in psychoanalytic therapy who is seriously concerned about the structure of his transference and relatedness, can be swayed by any presumptive posture his analyst takes—"behavior control machine," "spontaneous person" or anything else—since he is not ordinarily interested in entering into any psychological bargains, to purchase relief from his symptoms at the price of swallowing still another significant person's pretense about his role in relation to a patient. In short, this dispute fails to account for the overriding fact that a serious inquiry, to reveal some fundamental truth about a patient's experience, is far more useful than an analyst's decision about his "correct" attitude or posture in the therapeutic field. But, it may be countered, does this not beg the question that both the "behavior machine" and the "spontaneous person" are trying to answer? Is not the question, rather, how can an analyst best facilitate the emergence of such a psychological truth? In a word, by inquiry into the patient's problems. See, however, B. Wolstein, *Freedom to Experience*, New York: 1964, Part II.

that patterns of transference are recurrent, bound, automatic and beyond conscious awareness, they are readily predictable; but these are also the sort of characteristics the analyst looks for to define the operation of transferred distortions, and set the context of psychoanalytic inquiry. Beyond this, finally, are the effects of sheer will—of ornery willfulness, even—that have to be reckoned with. If, for example, a man claimed that two parts hydrogen and one part oxygen cannot be compounded as H_2O, the experimental chemist may simply ignore his opinion or, if he feels kindly disposed, refer him to a psychoanalytic consultant; if a man claimed that his present intolerance of frustration is not at all related to past parental indulgence, however, the analyst is obliged to listen to the facts of the case, because they may demonstrate a patient's belief about this integrative anomoly and about its generative conditions in his individual experience; yet, even after intensive inquiry, the establishment of this connection between intolerance of frustration and past parental indulgence still may not ring true until other of his unconscious defenses and beliefs have been worked through and reconstructed.

To penetrate directly to the patient's core, in such a case, requires the removal of his customary defenses from his reach: he has to be forced in some way to confront the repressed and unanalyzed structure of his basic personality and, when this challenging penetration succeeds, he is brought face to face with aspects of himself that he thus far has been able to avoid. As this approach forcibly pushes aside his unconscious defenses, his core problem and his core resources move into the foreground of the therapeutic field. But, then what? Presumably unconscious defenses are analyzed as unconscious resources are liberated. This, at least, is the idealized version of authoritarian psychoanalytic procedure. Once the patient is presumed capable of qualitatively new modes of relatedness, however, what becomes of the challenged defenses that authoritarian means force into the psychological background? These now are in the preconscious or unconscious sphere. The patient who willingly submits to this kind of therapeutic penetration, can elude the analyst's authoritarian procedure by retaining the distortion in a different form, and assigning it a different structural position so that it may persist undetected as a preconscious or unconscious process. Defensive projections have the character of a chameleon, and this dynamic character first prompted Freud, in spite of his pursuit of "military conquest," to abandon the hypnotic and pressure procedures very early in the history of psychoanalysis, even though he later failed to liberate psychoanalytic procedure from the therapeutic goals of these earlier procedures. But he did observe that a patient, undergoing hypnosis in order to resolve his symptomatology, transforms his psychic field of relatedness: the hypnotic trance does not remove defenses in response to the presumptive authority of the hypnotherapist, but simply moves them over the edges of the hypnotic focus. These defenses originally were derivative rather than central traumata; now, they remain unanalyzed, persisting beyond awareness and having effects in experiential fields for which they were not originally intended—so they become more troublesome as the hypnotherapist, this time, intervenes to remove them still further from their formative context.

These early observations of the effects of hypnotherapy on the patient's psychological field are clearly confirmed by the procedures of the authoritarian analyst. It remains impossible, by means of straight psychological analysis, to separate core structure from its derivative functions. Yet, this goal continues to attract a following, probably to satisfy recurrent yearnings for a radical simplification of the therapeutic process. Under present conditions of psychoanalytic inquiry, however, it is only an illusory possibility, formulated to justify undemonstrable metapsychological assumptions. This approach cuts and dries the analyst's task to fit the simplified requirements of a calculating automaton: routinely, he first separates structure from function, then mechanically analyzes appropriate aspects of structure to effect the desired changes, and finally withdraws to observe automatic changes in function—and, next patient, please! As he treats a basic structure without taking its derived functions into account, of course, its derived function becomes as unconscious and as unavailable as the now analyzed structure was originally, even though that particular structure may be mastered as a therapeutic result; for the original derived functions, after being forcibly removed from awareness, begin to take on the hardened qualities of psychic structure. No analyst, therefore, can freeze the movement of psychoanalytic process to keep both defensive function and repressed structure in the conscious foreground at one and the same time—not, at least, until their defensive and repressive qualities are analyzed when and as they appear. First of all, structure and function have different conditions of origin in the actual development of personality; second, they sustain the psychological identity of the patient's individuality in and through therapeutic change; third, and more generally, they uphold the forward moving continuity of psychic process. The authoritarian analyst, using methods of direct penetration, may help to reveal latent resources or, even, produce phenomenal gains on the basis of his patient's distorted transference—by an apparent flight to reality and to health but, in many cases, a flight from the analyst's authoritarianism—though still remaining to be analyzed are the relatively untouched defensive functions that such methods shunt out of therapeutic focus. These latter defenses will return to disturb the patient as new formations of repressed structure. The singular result of direct penetration is to make the patient even more defensive and, consequently, far less able than he originally was to perceive why he is still anxious and insecure. In itself, the complexity of this defensive system makes it self-defeating to begin psychoanalytic therapy at the directly intuited center of a patient's experience. If an analyst is sensitive, alert and tactful, he may eventually get there, but his direct intuitions usually attain their full sense and adequacy, empirically, as the psychoanalytic procedure evolves toward its terminal stages, only after the analysis of transference and resistance and of their convergence with countertransference and counterresistance has already been worked through.

The kernel of truth suggested by this authoritarian push for "core-to-core" experience is the centrality of psychological values it implies—the search for experience that is free of social facades, cultural constraints, familial anomolies or interpersonal pretenses a patient acquires in the course of his development, and that allows him, as he is, to look at himself fairly, squarely and relatedly. This is empirically a human potentiality because sociocultural and familial adjustments are not the whole man: there is, in addition, his private life of hope and aspiration, failure and disillusionment, joy and tragedy, but, then, neither is his private mode the whole man because it is continually being affected by the public conditions of its operation. Without a dynamic compenetration of the two, he would be a mechanical robot—at the mercy, in any event, of his unintegrated and underdeveloped behavior. Under these terms and conditions, his life may be rooted in biological nature, but he also responds imaginatively and reflectively to this and to other sectors of his natural environment. To deal with this rootedness in nature, though, he cannot just simply be: he must also become—acculturated and socialized in and by the heritage of interests, values and institutions to which he was born. And, mystical extentialism [3] to the contrary, his desire to know—understand, plan, act intelligently —is a trait as basic to his life experience as the useful distinction between his biology and his psychology and, in certain contexts of psychoanalytic inquiry, is even more useful. This desire to know is a fact of human nature that, as known and knowable, is not itself transcended.

Recent investigation has been organized about the hypothesis that psychoanalytic therapy is a shared experience, taking place within a common field of inquiry and involving the personalities of both analyst and patient.[4] The theories of transference and

[3] For this characterization of existentialism, see P. Tillich, "Existential Philosophy," *Journal of the History of Ideas*, V (1944), p. 67.

[4] For an early critique of the mirror conception of the analyst's role, see A. Balint and M. Balint, "On Transference and Countertransference," *International Journal of Psychoanalysis*, XX (1939), pp. 223–230. D. Lagache, "The Problem of Transference," in J. Frosch *et al.*, *Annual Survey of Psycho-*

resistance, to fit this perspective, have had to be reinterpreted; and since, in addition, the analyst's metapsychology no longer is privileged in the therapeutic field, any one communication about the meaning of life can become as important as any other in the evolution of the total process. With this enlarged view of the psychoanalytic process, the study of repressed feelings, thoughts and actions—quite unlike the method of authoritarianism or the metaphor of military operations—extends beyond the classical limits of oedipal experience, moving back and forth between the central problem and its derivative effects and over into unconscious resources to deal with them, and through various stages of personality development. The experiential field of therapy by design, therefore, provides the patient with opportunities to produce new and original meanings.

analysis, New York: 1952, suggested the analyst adopt attitudes of silence and passivity to induce frustration in the patient, ignoring how difficult it then becomes to distinguish transferred from original frustration. For reasons such as this, J. Spiegel, "The Social Roles of Doctor and Patient in Psychoanalysis and Psychotherapy," *Psychiatry,* XVII (1954), pp. 369–376, saw no way to interpret transference as a field phenomenon and therefore, was prepared to abandon it, altogether. However, see Chapter VII, above, pp. 100–122.

Once the relativity of transference and countertransference was generally accepted as an operating principle, of course, other sorts of problems arose about the actual therapeutic use of countertransference: for example, P. Greenacre, "The Role of Transference: Practical Considerations in Relation to Psychoanalytic Therapy," *Journal of the American Psychoanalytic Association,* II (1954), pp. 671–684, took the strict view of eliminating all relations with the patient other than the work of analysis; P. Heimann, "On Countertransference," *International Journal of Psychoanalysis,* XXXI (1950), pp. 81–84, recognized the therapeutic significance of countertransference reactions but hesitated to burden the patient with them; M. Little, "Countertransference and the Patient's Response to It," *International Journal of Psychoanalysis,* XXXII (1951), pp. 320–340, suggested using countertransference in its widest sense, however, as the analyst's total response; while E. Tauber and M. Green, *Prelogical Experience,* New York: 1959, and L. Tower, "Countertransference," *Journal of the American Psychoanalytic Association,* IV (1956), pp. 224–255, described how the analyst's involvement may actually contain and reflect his patient's problem; and B. Wolstein, *Countertransference,* New York: 1959, related transference and countertransference concretely to each other in terms of the experiential field of therapy in which they are observed to occur, and are capable of being analyzed.

To view a patient's experiential field as the active field or context in which new meanings are reconstructed out of old, and are later worked into behavior, is a difficult theme to pursue systematically because its empirical conditions have yet to be firmly defined in operational terms. Without rigidly adhering to old terminologies and without recklessly searching after new ones, however, exploratory efforts have the immediate utility of at least defrosting set usages for later reconstructions of theory. What about the rather complex issues, then, that arise from attempts to define therapeutic change? Questions immediately concern the conceptual force of adding such prefixes as "inter" and "intra" to "psychic" or "personal" as these now are being used in psychoanalytic inquiry: perhaps "psychic" or "personal" is as good therapeutically, or do they imply the notion of a self-enclosed and unrelated individual? Or, on the other hand, does the distinction of "interpersonal" and "intrapersonal" have to be preserved, in order to focus for clinical observation on what a purely "interpersonal" perspective, consistently applied, tends to gloss over? But if the "interpersonal" is surrendered, and its distinction from the "intrapersonal" loses its force, what becomes of clinical observations already made and gathered in the perspective of "interpersonal" theory? When these distinctions are set against the background of the principle of continuity, though, they become even more complicated. Are processes now observed to function "intrapersonally" to be described simply as such, or do they also have to be conceived in the context of "interpersonal" history? Or are processes now reported as being simply "personal" to be conceived as having emerged in full during psychoanalytic inquiry and as having been severed from their presumably tangled and complex "intrapersonal" origins? And what becomes of the future context of action—in line with established terminologies, perhaps best called "transpersonal" [5]—in which

[5] For a comparison of self-actional, interactional and transactional points of view, see J. Dewey and A. Bentley, *Knowing and the Known*, Boston: 1949; for comments on field or transactional theory applied to psychoanalytic inquiry, see B. Wolstein, *Freedom to Experience*, New York: 1964, Appendix.

new consequences are brought into being? The special import of a "transpersonal" specification of processes in the therapeutic field, aside from its obvious future reference, is that it helps to arrest any ineluctably "personal" process at the borders of the therapeutic field—any process, indeed, that lacks temporal dimensions like those of "intrapersonal" origin, "interpersonal" function or "transpersonal" expectation—since no psychoanalytic procedure deals systematically with purely "personal" introspections that are unaffected by the communications of others, or are unresponsive to conditions of relatedness in time and space.

Yet, the problem about ineluctably "personal" experience is more than the operational problem of managing an absolute egress from the conditions of human life and of still being able to tell the tale. It is more than the logical problem of infinite regress, as well, that led some observers back to the birth trauma for the sources of psychological disturbance,[6] and others even further back into the murky depths of the racial and collective unconscious to interpret human life.[7] It is, in fine, the substantive problem of whether and in what contexts it is possible to describe the basic stuff of human nature.[8] This, in brief, is how such lines of inquiry work: by adopting the introspective hypothesis, and applying it consistently, I am always free to affirm or to deny anything people say I am, or even anything I say I am, for only I can know by way of personal introspection and then assert who I am; but since, in fact, I can never be so absolutely certain of who I am that I can assert it now and forever and beyond any shadow of doubt, all introspective types of psychological analysis must finally come to terms with their deep roots in the Augustinian tradition of self-enlightenment, on the basis of which only God in the end knows or needs to know who I am—and whom,

6 See, for example, O. Rank, *Will Therapy, and Truth and Reality*, New York: 1945.

7 See, for example, C. Jung, *Contributions of Analytical Psychology*, New York: 1927.

8 For a statement of the current status of this problem, see G. Ryle, *The Concept of Mind*, London: 1949.

therefore, I must seek and believe in order even to know now what I thought I knew about myself. So, it is clear, use of the introspective method to support the validity of ineluctably "personal" processes is rarely direct or naïve, leading psychoanalytic inquiry away from its dominantly scientific concerns and, rigorously pursued, into a special type of theology—which is not above controversy in its own discipline. But ordinary psychoanalytic usage of this terminology, it is also clear, does not commit psychoanalytic procedure to the method or to any other aspect of Augustinian metaphysics. For though analysts may think of "introspection" during clinical inquiry to mean, for example, what the patient does when he "looks into himself," they would ordinarily limit their use of this term to their own descriptive and inferential operations that define his communications of and about his relatedness in a therapeutic field.

Thus, it is clear, even minor changes in conceptual terms often create as many problems as they are intended to resolve—which would be no drawback, in itself, so long as the problems are squarely faced, and the changes then sharpen the application of the whole conceptual scheme to empirical procedure. These theoretical intricacies would be even more embarrassing, however, if they did not actually point beyond the structure of psychoanalytic therapy to a major unsolved problem of contemporary civilization: the inconsistencies of individualism.[9] Yet, when the conditions of inquiry that ordinarily define psychoanalysis are ignored because they violate preferences in metapsychology, the therapeutic objective becomes even more difficult to attain, for the outlined differences among "intra-," "inter-" and "transpersonal" processes actually denote different aspects of experiential conditions in and through which a patient moves, to integrate his relationship with the analyst: "interpersonal" processes may be analyzed according to their integrative and disjunctive patterns as soon as the patient becomes aware of another person in his immediate field of experience; when that particular field is no

9 See B. Wolstein, *Irrational Despair*, New York: 1962, pp. 116–130, for further comments on this problem.

longer immediately present and as it later becomes part of his past, it joins his structure of "intrapersonal" processes, to be experienced as the funded effects of the now past "interpersonal" processes; but as that particular field is projected into his future context of living in terms of their judged probability and in terms of their felt desirability, its "transpersonal" character now consists of that expected state of affairs he hopes to enstate by reconstructing his relations to his current "interpersonal" field.[10] Without all three, however, a program and a procedure of psychoanalytic therapy are difficult to construct systematically or to apply consistently.

The existentialist view of immediate experience, for example, suggests that the experience of transference may be penetrated without acknowledging its existential origins or without integrating its existential effects. In this view of psychotherapy that seeks to replace the distinctive operations of psychoanalysis, its goal of direct insight turns the vital functions of transference, both genuine and distorted, into a dead end of psychic process— its definition trapping it within the circle of its own full immediacy—which is far too great a theoretical extinction to admit when carried out merely to reinforce the supratemporal notion of an unrelated and unintegrable sense of "I-am." [11] What actually results from this limited view of the self is a recurrent type of anxiety peculiar to existentialist analysis in which the self is

10 This statement of the issues is unfortunately complicated by a jawbreaking terminology, but psychoanalytic perspectives never seem to fade away. Though they may be sifted through, to select and define basic terms required for the organization of empirical inquiry, only the redundancies and duplications can be eliminated without damaging the essential core of theories and practices. For the reader who is not especially interested in the partisan defense of any particular metapsychology, to place these conditions of psychoanalytic inquiry in spatio-temporal continuity would suffice for the therapeutic relativity of transference and countertransference.

11 See, for example, M. Boss, *Psychoanalysis and Daseinanalysis*, New York: 1963, p. 32, for the attempt to remain as open as possible and to listen and see how man appears in his full immediacy. This may be desirable as an existentialist program; it is hardly possible as an existential event.

For an alternative view of immediacy as a relative distinction within expe-

compressed to remain enclosed within immediate walls of its absurdity, causing the eruption of existentialist anxiety. The main trouble with this view, however, is its programmatic neglect of the mediating functions of reflective intelligence to integrate the immediate experience of "I-am" with the rest of the organized personality, when and as it is achieved in and through its "intrapersonal" origins, "interpersonal" relations and "transpersonal" expectations. To retain the purity of this immediate ground of experience, and keep it from being contaminated by the alienated powers of science and technology, organizing and directive functions of the total personality are subordinated to attainment of full immediacy in the domain of existentialist analysis.

Worth considering, here, is the persistent confusion of conscious processes with their products in classical psychoanalytic theory, for existentialists have used this major weakness to justify their

rience, see H. Schneider, *Ways of Being,* New York: 1962; his usage suggests that it is confusing to speak of existential analysis or existential therapy when referring to the perspective now associated with Boss, Binswanger, van den Berg and so on. Theirs are existentialist perspectives; existence is the ordinary noun from which is derived the adjective, existential. This usage helps to penetrate confusions in semantics and confusions in fact: existentialism is thus one among many philosophies of existence; psychological therapies are all existential, while none need be existentialist in theory; or existentialist ontologies are not at all existential, they are abstract systems of ideas. J. Randall, Jr.'s *Nature and Historical Experience,* New York: 1958, contains other criticisms of existentialist ontologies, as well, while welcoming the concrete insights of individual existentialist writers.

Unclear usage of existentialist nomenclature has also led to repetitions of the classical psychoanalytic argument: it used to be said that everyone had a Freudian oedipus complex, and whoever denied it was unaware of its occurrence; now, it is being suggested that everyone living in this era is in fact an existentialist, and whoever denies it is also unaware of its truth. But are we all, indeed, unconscious existentialists? And if so, can all metapsychological differences among analysts be formulated in terms of existentialism? Beyond this, moreover, is the question of substantive gains from this translation of terminologies, especially since existentialist perspectives have yet to establish their claim to being valid alternatives to those now used in psychoanalytic inquiry.

separation of historical dimensions from dynamic psychology and from therapeutic procedure. This confusion is especially apparent when classical analysts, attempting a universal application of instinctual metapsychology, failed to hold contexts of interpretation clear and distinct under actual conditions of inquiry. Thus, for example, while the fact of transference may be considered universal in human experience, its myriad empirical manifestations as related to the beliefs and values of any individual human's experience are anything but universal since, out of the infinite varieties of concrete possibilities, every man synthesizes a unique cluster of qualities that in some sense is exclusively his own. Perhaps classical analysts, originally, were more interested in the widespread application of new metapsychological doctrines than in the firm foundation of empirical procedures and, therefore, ignored the lead of psychological observation that did not suit their theoretical purposes.

The asserted universality of Freud's oedipal theory, furthermore, makes it practically impossible to determine just what sort of clinical evidence he required to establish it as definitive in the individual case. Since, moreover, there are dimensions of childhood experience that cannot be forced under purely libidinal and aggressive ones, the elevation of any monism or dualism to the level of a first principle is, at best, only arbitrary—more a deadly indictment of the standard conventions of Freud's environing culture than a universal principle of psychoanalytic inquiry. But his oedipal theory still might have earned universal status had he expanded its meaning to cover the plural phases of child development, in which all infants are born into familial settings as helpless, dependent, undifferentiated, in need of acculturation —no matter how societies set specific conditions for the structure and organization of its families. What these phases of development then mean for any individual child, is to be decided only by the empirical study of his particular history, since assignment of behavioral values and nurture of developmental values vary from culture to culture, from family to family within a single subculture and, from time to time, even within the same family. To propose, in other words, that every infant is born into a socially defined matrix of the family is one thing, and there probably is no disagreement about this practically self-evident proposition; but to assert that a complex oedipal phase of sexual development emerges in the childhood of everyone's experience through a pre-figured patterning of libido that follows its own course irrespec-tive of specific psychological environments with parents and other significant adults, siblings and preschool playmates, or classmates and teachers, is an entirely different sort of proposition. How-ever, the two are easily confused in a theory of psychoanalytic inquiry that, as a standard practice, attempts to universalize the meaning of clinical observations and to make all individual cases fit its predetermined scheme.

In spite of these difficulties, classical analysis already has a large niche in the history of modern psychology. Its position is secure, now, in part because post-Freudians have made many basic revi-sions in its theory and practice, in part because its metapsychol-ogy did not obscure any central observations of structures and functions of the human psyche under clinical inquiry. Perhaps crudely at first, but nonetheless empirically, it began to outline the processes of transference, resistance, free association and his-tory—as converging and correlative processes in a structured field of therapeutic inquiry. Only on this groundwork, moreover, was it later possible to observe and interpret the concomitant recur-rence of anxiety and distortion, the genuine and the distorted aspects of transference, or the relativity of transference and coun-tertransference. Had classical analysis consistently followed the distinction between psychology and metapsychology—empirically observable processes of consciousness, that is, and their concrete products of belief and value in action—it would now have been the reconstructed base of contemporary psychoanalysis.[12] Crowd-

12 Attempting to rectify this, the most recent codifier of classical analysis, D. Rapaport, in "The Structure of Psychoanalytic Theory," *Psychological Issues*, II (1960) , pp. 1-158, sharply distinguished the structure of psychoanaly-tic theory from the structure of psychoanalytic therapy, defining the basic method of psychoanalysis as that of interpersonal relation (p. 125) yet, at the

ing wide variations of fact into cramped uniformities of theory, classical analysis stopped short of studying the actual therapeutic field as constituted by two quite individual personalities who never so resemble one another that their histories and values— in short, their metapsychologies—coincide; instead, it erroneously approached both participants in the therapeutic field as self-enclosed systems of value that were the same through and through —interpretive speculation, sometimes fanciful, often stretched, made them so—when, in fact, they were far more similar with respect to their psychological processes of integration and dissociation. Nor did it adapt its therapeutic procedure to the knowledge that the analyst who, in theory, accepts the ultimacy of such differences in history and value, in practice enlarges his own observational range of his patient's power to move and to grow. The vision was, no doubt, noble—to start from biology, and construct a universal human psychology—but it turned sour when special repressions of a particular subculture were read back into the basic structure of human nature and, as metapsychology, treated like the principles of biology. It was not recognized, unfortunately, that metapsychology could never become a general science whose principles had the same validity as those of biology or psychology. This is the point where classical analysis over-stepped the boundaries of science, and entered the domain of philosophy and values—to express the spirit of an era or, perhaps, just reflect the passing fads of popular fancy.

Under the circumstances, classical insistence on a thoroughgoing psychic determination no longer is convincing.[13] It is potentially misleading, furthermore, in suggesting that a process

same time, describing the theoretical propositions of the system independently of accumulated clinical evidence (p. 111)—there being, in his view, no canon to distinguish valid interpretation from pure speculation during clinical inquiry (p. 112).

13 See C. Brenner, *An Elementary Textbook of Psychoanalysis*, Garden City: 1955, and D. Rapaport, "The Structure of Psychoanalytic Theory," *Psychological Issues*, II (1960), pp. 1–158, for current restatements of this principle.

or event, rather than a theory about certain properties of that process or event, can be said to be deterministic. The principle that from a select number of metapsychological variables all aspects of experience are fully and accurately predictable, that chance and novelty are of no effect or consequence, that variations and dimensions of experience cannot actually occur—the doctrine, in brief, of historical inevitability—here is being called determinism. This principle, above all others, has provided the foundation in metapsychology for the absolute certainty that classical analysts seek to reproduce in their practice. But it held out far more promise in theory than it ever could deliver in fact, thereby complicating the cumulative record of transference and countertransference in therapeutic transaction with distorted images of omniscience and omnipotence. Steeped in the mechanistic determinism of nineteenth-century science, history and philosophy, classical analysts would have to strain for a looser yet more accurate notion like historical conditioning that suffices, today, for the psychoanalytic study of psychological change. While some interpreters carefully couch their Freudianism in the language and logic of its originator,[14] the conceptual innovations of twentieth-century science and philosophy have compelled others to reconsider the whole classical framework, especially to rework its biological metapsychology so as to return personality to the sociocultural and interpersonal conditions of its development and function.[15] Because of disagreement over these conceptual inno-

---

[14] For example, H. Hartmann, "Technical Implications of Ego Psychology," *Psychoanalytic Quarterly*, XX (1951), pp. 31–43; E. Kris, "Ego Psychology and Interpretation in Psychoanalytic Therapy," *Psychoanalytic Quarterly*, XX (1951), pp. 15–30; and R. Loewenstein, "The Problem of Interpretation," *Psychoanalytic Quarterly*, XX (1951), pp. 1–14. But, compare S. Hook (ed.), *Psychoanalysis, Scientific Method and Philosophy*, New York: 1959.

[15] See E. Fromm, *Escape from Freedom*, New York: 1941; F. Fromm-Reichmann, *Principles of Intensive Psychotherapy*, Chicago: 1950; K. Horney, *The Neurotic Personality of Our Time*, New York: 1937; H. Sullivan, *Conceptions of Modern Psychiatry*, Washington: 1947; C. Thompson, *Psychoanalysis*, New York: 1950.

vations, or through adherence to ritualized performance, the original problems of classical theory continue to overshadow the enduring and valuable kernel of psychoanalytic discoveries. Psychic determinism is a prime example of the sort of unworkable principle that hinders scientific growth in psychoanalysis: in the therapeutic field, it materially affects neither the operational analysis of causation nor the historical study of psychological events—except, of course, when the analyst introduces it as part of his conceptual frame of reference—since the formulation of a causal nexus, no matter how extensive the accumulated information, is at best tentative, provisional and open to change in the light of new empirical observation. To determine earlier causes of later outcomes in the context of active inquiry, moreover, requires the controlled specification of initial conditions under which the inquiry is undertaken. This postulate of scientific empiricism has no metatheoretical status apart from the varieties of inquiry that are organized and controlled by it. When an inquiry succeeds, though, it succeeds empirically and results in the reliable description of sequences of cause and effect without, however, ascribing an inherent determinism to them. The notion that every effect has its cause is a necessary one: it acquires logical validity through the operational definition of cause and effect; but this notion is also an empirical one that can be used to establish recurrent relations of antecedents and consequents in carefully controlled observation. From this it may be concluded that, in psychoanalytic uses of determinism, extrascientific commitments far outweigh scientific ones.

In spite of heavy reliance on historical methods, classical analysis fails to deal with the cumulative continuity of experience as it moves forward. In id therapy, the meaning and use of history are freighted with a reductive, mechanistic determinism. Appreciation of this fact would temper the harsh, often misfired criticisms that are leveled against psychoanalysis by those who lack first hand knowledge of its empirical observations; its findings are not accepted by philosophers on the grounds of unclear systematic usage and unanchored metapsychological speculation; nor are its procedures well regarded by experimental psychologists who work with the overt behavior of animals. These critics have yet to appreciate the powerful impetus behind the psychoanalytic enterprise, however, since Breuer and Freud and into the present. Freud, for example, was willing to look everywhere, despite the severe limitations of his inherited philosophy of science, in his effort to understand the structure of experience. The most enduring result of his search was that he expanded the procedural range of psychological inquiry in a face to face situation. Yet, he was also prepared to treat everything as intelligible and nothing, at the outset, as sacrosanct and as beyond rational scrutiny—major and minor pathologies of everyday life, hypnotic phenomena and conversion symptoms, dreams and jokes, slips of the tongue and dissociated body movements, transference and resistance, individual history and familial environment, literature and mythology, cultural history and archeology, social ritual and social organization, anthropology and religion—in fact he made all experience his proper domain. Unfortunately, strict application of a narrow instinctual determinism during his later years obstructed his interpretive vision. When a man sets out, however, to encompass the whole universe of psychological events—in itself a hazardous but courageous undertaking—the scope of his imagination is at least remarkable for the attempt, especially because of the stubborn and fateful foreknowledge that he is bound to fail. Freud, of course, was driven by an extraordinary singularity of purpose—to establish the universal application of his metapsychology of personality, and support it with the principle of psychic determinism—and his was the mammoth task of reducing the manifold of experience and of fitting it into a mechanical repetition of past events, in order to validate eros and thanatos as his first causes. At the same time, though, he precluded the ongoing present and anticipated future from his theory of therapy and, as a result, neglected such themes as the relation of transference and anxiety in the forward movement of therapeutic communication, the unconscious convergence of transference and countertransference in current fields of therapeutic inquiry, and the reconstructive judgments of attitude and behavior whose chief points of reference still are in the unlived future.

But classical analysts are not alone. Some who seek the philosophic union of psychoanalysis and moral theory have yet to distinguish their own principles of psychology from that of psychic determinism in classical psychoanalytic theory.[16] Any advance at all in this direction, of course, represents a significant advance in philosophic inquiry, but special difficulties arise because the classical psychoanalysis of unconscious processes is invoked to defend a moral determinism that was probably affirmed prior to the discovery of this new psychology. For these writers seem to subscribe to the rather awkward notion that the more an individual learns about his history, the less he may be held responsible for the course of his current conduct; and the individual who reached the ideal limit of full self-knowledge presumably could live without responsibility, on the ground that his actions are driven by factors and forces outside his controlling awareness. A crucial instance is the moral agent who cannot be held responsible for his current actions because he could not do otherwise, since he lacks control over the original shaping of his character. He is, therefore, not responsible for acting the way he does, on the further assumption that the original factors that shape his character are now major determinants of its current workings. This line of reasoning is deterministic: that he could not have done otherwise, that origins and aims of his behavior are patterned independently of one another, and that every process runs its course to predetermined conclusions unaffected by any other in the psychic domain. Hence, the dilemma of the consistent determinist in psychology or morals: once he decides that no agent can be held responsible for predetermined conduct, whom does he then hold responsible, not to hold the agent responsible? But the breakdown of belief in determinism during psychoanalytic inquiry is far more poignant and far more significant therapeutic-

16 See S. Hook (ed.), *Psychoanalysis, Scientific Method and Philosophy*, New York: 1959, for example, pp. 336–357.

ally than the breakdown of its logical consistency, for the notion that patients can now be only what past external conditions allow them to become, aside from turning felt experience into a passive mass of stoic suffering, may itself become a rationalization for hopelessness and empty defeat, for boredom and aimless despair.

In psychoanalytic inquiry, patients often appeal to determinism after making frankly self-defensive appraisals of ingrained and crippling disabilities, in order to attribute them directly to this or that actual or imagined event in early childhood. They first construe themselves as having been the passive victim of another's irrational behavior, usually at or around the age of five; then they ascribe great explanatory power to its uncanny hold on post-childhood experience. What they overlook, so long as they do not worship at the deterministic altar of past history, is that no two situations so pointedly correspond as to prevent felt nuances and environed factors from emerging to make a change possible. Chiefly because stories about a cruel childhood fate are not questioned in psychoanalytic determinism, are they invoked to explain patently unrelated events of later life. Why patients fail to become aware of significant differences, however, becomes a central therapeutic issue; and intensive study of the actual situations in which that early event is resurrected to justify later conduct reveals far more about its current unconscious meaning than it does about its original impact, as it can now be recalled. What the early event presumably explains in current conduct, moreover, is often capable in its own right of producing anxiety and guilt—the pressure to explain suggesting that these determinists already accept far more responsibility than they care to acknowledge; but they take a once meaningful, now isolated pattern or event, and make of it perfunctory exercises so as to disown responsibility for their current conduct. Acceptance of this responsibility, they seem to recognize, involves a serious search for ways and means of reconstructing the conditions of its presumed recurrence; instead, they devote their energies to the security and fleeting comfort of immediatized and rationalized defenses. Yet, no experience is comprehensible or changeable so long as its subject remains motionless or monotonous.

Psychoanalysis, however else construed, is still a study of psychological change, and for this reason, as well, appeals to determinism are often made in the face of procedural inadequacies to shore up faltering convictions about the value of psychological inquiry. From the uneven success of current procedures with certain pathological conditions, however, no immutable laws about their intrinsic nature can be inferred. To convert current defects of therapeutic procedure into deterministic principles of metapsychology, therefore, is but an empty gesture—except, perhaps, that the deterministic hypothesis is a sad cloak for ignorance. If classical analysts are practically convinced about psychic determinism, to be consistent they should discontinue therapeutic efforts at intervention in the lives of their patients, just as philosophic determinists should long since have discontinued their efforts at a sound moral theory. Instead, they might both counsel passive acquiescence to a characterological fate. Determinism and pessimism thus go hand in hand, but a true pessimism fails even to generate professions of determinism. And this is the vital blindspot of all determinisms in psychology and morals: without a sense of personal response and responsibility, the psychological power of knowledge is neutralized.

Still another aspect of this issue concerns the creation of a permissive, nonjudgmental atmosphere in the therapeutic field so that patients may more openly reveal themselves. Because the psychoanalytic determinist considers this highly significant for carrying out his procedure, he first reinforces it with the systematic distinction of the normal from the abnormal on a quantitative basis—as distinct, again, from the qualitative stuff of the human psyche that is held common to all men—and then articulates and expands it at levels of theory far removed from therapeutic experience with the severely disturbed conditions that he frequently cites to support his conceptual scheme. Accordingly, the bizarre communications of schizophrenic patients only appear to be qualitatively unique because of their idiosyncratic use of language, logic and gesture. Their extreme attempts at individual productivity represent, instead, quantitative failures in the growing process of individuation, and such clinical individualism in the extreme is actually a hollow caricature of the person they may yet become. This, of course, is one result of the fallacy of misplaced abstractness for, in psychological fact, qualities are no less analyzable than quantities. Though these patients act, then, as if their sense of self were highly differentiated out of a solid base, they meanwhile are genuinely helpless and terrified, their psychological growth threatening to become atrophied. They tend to project exaggerated expressions of a still unfound self in order to convince analyst and significant others in their immediate environment—and themselves, as well—that they have something unique and unrealized that is worth intensive psychological effort. But they are painfully dependent upon positive responses to this self-dramatization; they are pressured to communicate increasingly bizarre material, hoping to call attention to their crippling disturbances.

Following the principle of determinism and its corollary—namely, that changes in quantity accompanying changes in quality define disturbances in relatedness—the analyst who then ignores his patient's qualitative impact in its own terms, thereby does not confirm the principle or its corollary. He has, in fact, adopted a rule of procedure to provide his patient with the experiential latitude for bringing previously unconscious patterns and potentialities into therapeutic focus, hoping that both he and his patient will become better acquainted with them. As a rule, this procedure is designed to enable the patient to learn how he came to be what he really is, or what he believes himself to have become, in the previously unknown sectors of his total personality. Such an exploration, however, does not illustrate the axiomatic relation of quality and quantity any more than it illustrates the principle of psychoanalytic determinism. For procedures of inquiry still are not postulates of metapsychology, and this is why they do not explain away a patient's responsibility for his current conduct. In any event, there is a point reached in therapeutic inquiry at which the distinction of quantity and quality becomes superfluous in principle—at which differences in degree no longer reflect significant correlations, and differences in kind no longer produce significant changes.

In the short history of psychoanalysis, wrong metapsychology has frequently contributed to the undoing of an otherwise right therapy. Whenever, indeed, an analyst's belief about any principle of metapsychology is raised to the level of absolute conviction, it confuses his steady observation of the therapeutic field. Its protracted use hopelessly entangles the described material he selects for inference with unobserved effects of his metapsychology. Then, of course, as the patient presents material that verifies his analyst's absolutes, both tend to ignore marginal or negative material and, as a consequence, cause it to be altered and extended out of its original context of meaning. Beyond these difficulties is the unconscious tendency to accept beliefs about relatively unknown or unexplored phenomena, and follow them without question because they appear more profound in the absence of clear verifiability or because they are endorsed by charismatic authorities. In conceptions of therapeutic inquiry, Freud's theory of instincts and Jung's notion of archetypes are examples of inappropriate mediating terms of procedure: the one was as mythological as the other was supernatural. Conceptions of the same order, however, are also found in the psychologies of existentialist and mystical analysis, if only because their negative attitudes toward science and technology encourage the development of abstract theories that have no practical relevance—but much critical work has already been devoted to the inadequacies of all these frameworks of psychoanalytic inquiry.[17]

[17] For example, see B. Apfelbaum, *Dimensions of Transference in Psychotherapy*, Berkeley & Los Angeles, 1958; F. Fromm-Reichmann, *Principles of Intensive Psychotherapy*, Chicago: 1950; R. Grinker *et al.*, *Psychiatric Social Work*, New York: 1961; S. Hook (ed.), *Psychoanalysis, Scientific Method and Philosophy*, New York: 1959; E. Schachtel, *Metamorphosis*, New York: 1959; E. Tauber and M. Green, *Prelogical Experience*, New York: 1959; C. Thompson, *Psychoanalysis*, New York: 1950; and B. Wolstein, *Irrational Despair*, New York: 1962.

A more recent attempt at theory—the notion of biogenetic pleasure[18]—has escaped this sort of critical attention, even though its construction is especially disconcerting in a psychoanalytic approach that follows the tradition of scientific naturalism. As part of a general theory of psychodynamics, this notion represents a serious attempt to deal with observable process. Any such biogenetic interpretation of pleasure during actual therapy, however, pushes the empirical evidence outside the domain of psychological inquiry. It lends strong support, moreover, to those traditional habits of thought that acknowledge the self-sustaining validity of psychological inquiry so long as it produces the desired results. Is it but a present-day recurrence of the neurologizing tautology that prevailed in late nineteenth-century conceptions of psychopathology and that now reappears in biological terms? If, indeed, this notion of biogenetic pleasure is a biologizing tautology, it is hardly relevant at the explanatory level to the structure of psychoanalytic therapy. Yet, during therapeutic inquiry, its interpretive use as a defensive rationalization is far more relevant: appeals to the notion of biogenetic defect may easily obstruct the serious adaptational patient's quest for active psychological conditions of pleasure and pain. Faced with his analyst's theory that locates the problem in biology and genetics, he is back where he started, again alone with his own resources and having to discover those psychological conditions on his own. Evidently, this adaptational theory is well adapted to the prejudgments and prejudices of its environing culture, in respect to its obstructive effects on the unfolding therapeutic inquiry. Even prior to inquiry, it erects a biogenetic barrier to the steady observation of psychological processes by which, alone, a patient may expand his scope of awareness, clarity of knowledge and range of action, in having experiences of pleasure. Let the biologist, the neurologist, the physician tell him the actual biological limits of his capacity to experience when and as they can; let the

[18] S. Rado, "Dynamics and Classification of Disordered Behavior," *American Journal of Psychiatry*, CX (1953), pp. 406–424.

psychiatrist, the psychologist, the psychotherapist attempt inquiry to define the experiential limits of his capacities for pleasure; and no matter how a neuropsychiatrist joins the results of both fields of inquiry, let the patient draw his own conclusions, finally, about the limits of his own experience when he bumps into them and as they become, literally, objective.[19] By predefining the limits of individual psychoanalytic inquiry, then, this notion of biogenetic pleasure already prepares for a sense of deprivation and failure before the psychotherapeutic work is done. Since it may serve only to cushion a sensed failure about using the psychoanalytic instruments to their fullest, its proponents might explore the limitations of the instruments themselves, for this knowledge is far more useful than the construction of still another metapsychology in the traditional psychoanalytic manner.

Even though a definition of pleasure in terms of gene, absurdity, libido or archetype, when spelled out empirically, could support a theory of individual differences in psychoanalytic therapy, these terms often set premature limits to the practical explorations of an individual patient's experience. This does not mean, of course, that objective limits do not exist—because, in fact, they do —but, rather, that limits have to be derived empirically, in accordance with the actual conditions of each individual and within a perspective that openly extends into a partly defined, partly undefined future. If the analyst even temporarily surrenders absolute terms of metapsychology, he then is free to follow the experiential thread that actually evolves in the therapeutic field —beginning with the emergence of his patient's anxiety and, within the context of his own countertransference, observing a pattern of increasing anxiety as a direct response to his intruding

[19] See R. Sobel, "Role Conflict or Resistance," *American Journal of Psychotherapy*, XVIII (1964), pp. 25–34, for a clear description of how the role of the psychiatric patient differs from that of the medical patient, demanding opposite kinds of behavior from both participants. Just as confusion of roles by doctor and patient may be the source of some transferred resistances, it may also be the source of some countertransferred counterresistances.

concerns about his own metapsychology. It would be obstructive, however, for the analyst to continue pushing an abstract meta-theory—assuming in advance that every patient can be understood only in terms of his special theory—and, meanwhile, ignoring its immediate effects on the unfolding therapeutic inquiry. The structure of psychoanalytic therapy is, first and last, a structure of inquiry: it has no special philosophy of life to sell; and it hardly is a new preachment in secular theology.

Not unlike this biogenetic notion, on the other hand, is the use of communication theory to interpret the therapeutic experience of psychoanalysis, reducing its qualitative richness and diversity to a series of linear communication networks. One exponent of communication theory has explicitly developed this point: "My model enables us to study, and . . . to relate cultural to social events; it is ideally suited to the purpose. It is not suited for studying pathology, because the question raised in studying pathology is not answered by that sort of model . . . my model is essentially bound to the study of signals, impulses, messages—whatever you want to call them. If you deal with things in which the impulse or message is excluded, this model is no good." [20] Objective models of communication theory have limited value in the study of psychopathology because, in short, they do not deal with unconscious aspects of relatedness and communication, of transference and resistance. Excluded from therapeutic inquiry, as well, are all immediate, directly felt aspects of experience, since these models are about questions like who talks to whom? about what? under what conditions? with what message? to what effect?—overlooking, however, the direct feelings of the communication and their meaning for further psychic integration. But this communication theory is no less questionable than is, say, the existentialist withdrawal from the reflective complex-

---

[20] J. Ruesch, "The Observer and the Observed: Human Communication Theory," in R. Grinker (ed.), *Toward a Unified Theory of Human Behavior*, New York: 1956, p. 50. By permission of Basic Books, Inc.

ities of a patient's experience.[21] Strictly applied, both suffer from the same defect; oppositely, they narrow the psychoanalytic field by severing a patient's therapeutic network of communication from his others, in this way seeking to reduce anxiety and to liberate the flow of repressed information. But the information might just as well remain repressed since, in the communication model, it becomes available for study without explicit reference to feelings or purposes. Thus, aspects of communication that can be studied by this analyst will remain detached from his patient's experiential relation to them. Repressing what transcends the sheltered boundaries of this procedure, moreover, the patient then has to explore unconscious therapeutic relations on his own —if, of course, he can—or find himself a different kind of analyst.

A frequent argument for standardizing psychoanalytic inquiry, even to the point of making up psychocomputer syndromes, is the systematic and mathematical precision with which it minimizes or eliminates fallibilities of human judgment from the analyst's response to his patient. The mathematical analyst's effort to compute his patient's communications also suppresses and represses communications that do not fit the machines which, in turn, tend to induce special types of anxiety and distortion as conditioned results of failing to attend to these suppressions and repressions.

[21] Ruesch, for example, exhibits this very neatly: in communication theory, he can be scientific but not about distorted experience (R. Grinker (ed.), *Toward a Unified Theory of Human Behavior*, New York: 1956, p. 50); with distorted experience, he cannot use communication theory or be scientific about it (L. Salzman and J. Masserman (eds.), *Modern Concepts of Psychoanalysis*, New York: 1962, p. 91).

This central problem of the relation of science and experience, curiously enough, is shared by the communication and the existentialist analysts, both locked in dispute over "spontaneous" immediatism or "behavior control" science yet neither able to get beyond the dualism they also assert about the felt and the known. Hence, their common dilemma about the problem of values in psychoanalytic therapy (see, above, p. 228, footnote 2). But this dualism of the felt and the known need not be taken as a generic trait of human being —not, at least, until its cultural and philosophic roots have been more thoroughly explored in current habits of thinking and patterns of living.

This is scientific approach, according to the psychocomputer's argument, reliably scientific. But is it? The experience of most psychoanalytic patients does not fit the computer patterns of communication analysis—the psychopathic and bizarre, shy and unmotivated, rebellious and iconoclastic, underdeveloped and overprivileged—those, in other words, who benefit most from a psychological analysis of their relatedness and communication. It is still impossible, in any case, to translate distorted and genuine patterns, emotional and reflective probabilities, unexpressed and still novel possibilities, into a numerical and programmed analysis that is meaningful and useful. Beyond this, moreover, is the most troublesome thing about psychoanalytic procedure by computer in terms of linguistics and communication—which, of course, is not the same as making the results of psychoanalytic therapy compatible with communication theory for purposes, say, of interdisciplinary research: inevitably, this analyst tends to gear his therapeutic work, not to the individual needs, securities and fulfillments of his patients but to the conditions and classifications of programming their communications; in other words, the judgment of an impersonal mechanism is tacitly substituted for the experience of the analyst himself actually judging the experience of his patient. Especially disconcerting, however, are those therapeutic fields in which the patient is capable of originality— new feeling, new meaning, new pattern—but, instead, must carefully train himself to meet requirements that are set by the tested significance of psychocomputer analysis. Research analysts, as well, are forced to avoid experimental programs of therapy under special conditions unless they can forge obvious linkages with that model of communication theory.

In order, for these reasons, is a reappraisal of the push to modify established models of psychoanalytic inquiry, and append them to general systems theory or to unified behavior theory, since psychoanalysis so far has gained little from mechanical standardizations. The presumption of such hard and fast objectivity in the therapeutic field is chiefly supported by a blank wall of detachment, without regard for the immediate pressures of a patient's feelings, or the future of his active purposes. With the classical mirror so mechanized, the special psychoanalytic field of communication is capable of being related only to other equally special extrapsychoanalytic fields of communication. And with no regard for the patient's thrust of will, no analyzed pattern can be observed to extend beyond its already defined fields of communication. Whenever any operational scheme rests its case exclusively on the results of psychocomputer analysis, its perspective fails to consider precarious, accidental, unplanned and impressionistic qualities of felt experience. Nor does it effectively describe the emergent processes of personal change: it certainly cannot deal with them in the round, as live events. At best, finally, it may provide guides, probes and profiles of a general sort; it cannot replace the shared experience and analysis of transference and countertransference, by now a well established condition of psychoanalytic therapy.

Thus, two superficially opposed views of the structure of psychoanalytic inquiry, communication theory and existentialist analysis, unexpectedly converge in their actual impact on the shared experience of the therapeutic field. To much the same effects, reliance on extreme objectivity confines and distorts the analyst's practical functions as does his reliance on the extreme subjectivity of "I-am": the communicational and the existentialist analysts adopt anonymous roles as a rule of procedure so as to curtail the effects of their transactions, respectively, on a patient's private system of communication or on his private experience of "I-am." Yet, in spite of such ostensible wishes to avoid interfering, the private flow of experience ordinarily has little worth apart from the needs, goals and ideals to which it points, and it is practically worthless to the aloof analyst who has withdrawn from therapeutic involvement. Explicit concern with imaginative fantasies is still valid, though, even if these are apparently produced to satisfy the analyst's participating requirements; and, of course, there still is no substitute for the discipline, dedication and courage to work fantasies through to realizations. But the analyst's anonymity may easily spread beyond the immediate therapeutic field, and serve to protect his patient with new ways of avoiding the things that matter in his everyday life; by adopting this same facade of anonymity, a patient may also avoid the fears and anxi-eties about things that matter, and shield himself, as well, against defensive lethargy and destructive cynicism—a prevalent pattern of the bored, the depressed and the schizoid who so frequently are at present seen in the private practice of psychoanalytic ther-apy. What is missing from these perspectives, then, is open acknowledgement of the importance of what ails the patient and of how a direct personal experience can help to effect a mutative transaction—without which, of course, therapy would be an exer-cise in psychological gymnastics, putting some new wrinkles into theory but avoiding any new muscles in action.

Though these doctrines have been defended as presumptive answers to the moral crisis of our time, they actually threaten any possible general rapprochement of science and human values; in fact, they endanger the considerable efforts already exerted to construct a coherent structure of psychonalytic therapy. If, they argue, analysts reject the transformation of their role into a "behavior control machine," and do not succumb to the irra-tional temper of mysticism, they will fall heir to the quiescent despair of existentialism. But, of course, since mysticism and existentialism do not advance formulations of psychotherapy enough to justify abandoning hard won positions of psycho-analysis, it becomes appropriate to understand why these doc-trines have cropped up in recent discussion. And they are curious developments because, at least since the turn of the century, psychoanalytic psychology has been firmly rooted in the tradi-tions of science, while modifications and enlargements of its pro-cedures have been guided by traits of its subject matter that dis-tinguish it from other domains of science. Ordinarily, philoso-phers of science ascribe to the structure of science and to the terms and conditions of its procedures, the standards of precision, reliability, objectivity, simplicity and comprehensiveness.[22] On

22 See E. Nagel, *The Structure of Science*, New York: 1961, and H. Feigl, "Some Major Issues and Developments in the Philosophy of Science of Logical Empiricism," in H. Feigl and M. Scriven (eds.), *The Foundations of Science and the Concepts of Psychology and Psychoanalysis*, Minneapolis: 1956.

the basis of this general model, they then treat psychoanalysis as unscientific essentially because its subject matter prevents it from fully realizing these standards with the conventional clarity of other established sciences. As a result, some conclude, it is placed beyond the pale—with every other type of inquiry, of course, that does not satisfy the operational requirements of mathematico-experimental methods—and they withhold the scientific designation. Yet, mysticism and existentialist analysis also conform to this fairly conventional view and readily surrender the scientific status of psychoanalysis. These also separate the rationality of physical nature from the irrationality of human nature, raising serious doubts about any intelligible ordering of psychological events; their dualism precludes any further scientific structuring of psychoanalytic inquiry. In experience as in values, however, the notion of intelligible order among human events implies at least the possibility of a scientific psychology. Otherwise, it is futile and pointless even to try being rational about human problems. No mystic or existentialist can in fact adopt this extreme, though logical, extention of his premises and, at the same time, remain a sound therapist: he has to forsake his theory, if only to the extent of reacting creatively and intelligently to human problems as they become evident and intelligible in the therapeutic field.

When, therefore, an existentialist analyst seeks conditions of pure insight during therapeutic inquiry, after first attaining the experience of "I-am" and then leaping into absolute being, he has to proceed from these existentialist goals to actual significance in everyday life. He still has to face the unanswered questions about his exercise of existentialist analysis—why the struggle to undergo it, and what to do with its results once attained. No doubt difficult to answer, these questions remain unasked in his point of view—which one leading spokesman, as already noted,[23] terms mysticism—and the patient who takes it seriously and follows it religiously, is forced to drop central aspects of his personality from therapeutic inquiry so as to fit himself to patterns of exist-

23 See, above, p. 232, reference footnote 3.

entialist being. When an existentialist analyst thus experiences or observes the integration of insight, he remains ever dubious about its sources and about its aims—since absurd immediacy, after all, neither requires rational insight for itself nor generates any by itself; the existentialist patient need never attempt to judge, evaluate, appraise, understand or simply note, even, the content and direction of his immediate experience but, instead, may continue to drift with the confused and purposeless flux of his immediacy. It is by now a truism, perhaps, that emotion may be examined as well as lived; yet, no matter how fully the existentialist feels or how consistently he lives his feeling, failure to determine the appropriate conditions for examining emotion is no less self-destructive than failure to have immediate awareness of emotion. He may actually distort nonreflective aspects of experience by adopting a narrow framework that fails to relate them to reflection. If, as he moves through the immediate foreground of his experience, he has the freedom at least to inquire about its meaning, he may again discover why the unexamined life still is an unlived life. But where he represses reflective intelligence, and when he enforces this repression by an elaborate ontological wall, he can make no attempt at the exploration of confused emotion. In phenomenological terms, the existentialist self not only cannot become an object of its rational understanding; it no longer is even the subject of its own immediate experience.

It is difficult, therefore, to generate enthusiasm for the use of absolute immediatism in psychoanalytic therapy. The existentialist analyst has yet to free his formulations of the transcendental cobwebs that obscure the common ground of experience that is occupied by both reason and emotion. These integral traits of experience can offer one another something of worth only when neither drowns its identity in absolute communion with the other. They are not dissolved into pure being as simple fulfillment of wish; nor, indeed, are they forced to go away by a simple assertion of will. Lost in commitment to absolute immediatism, the existentialist analyst can salvage very little from the historical values of science, art or philosophy. After taking brief and uncharted flights into the stratosphere of existentialist immediacy, he returns to the "here and now" with the astonishing revelation that rhythmic burpings of the human infant demonstrate a more perfect union with the ultimate ground of being than does all adult experience—which, by definition, is warped because it is capable of becoming self-directively rational, hence alienated, about itself.

There is no clear way to explore motives underlying existentialist formulations of psychoanalysis. Explored within a therapeutic field, of course, the outline of their motivational matrix is more reliable than any drawn by pure speculation. Yet, clearly, no such therapeutic inquiry is essential to the systematic analysis of existentialist principles. Nor, in fact, are the systematic and procedural defects of any philosophical psychology to be identified with the personal psychology of its spokesmen. Psychogenetic analysis of ideas along the lines of individual unconscious psychology does not ordinarily produce better understanding of systematic formulations or procedural rules anyway—though it may in the future, perhaps, under ideal and purified conditions that still are beyond empirical possibility. The line now separating ideal from idealized conditions of inquiry remains incredibly thin, and since no one is so aware of all his biases in scientific judgment that he can certainly refrain from crossing it, the history and biography of ideas are to be sharply distinguished from their systematic validity and from their empirical application. Biography may illuminate the psychology of ideas, but biography itself is then ideas about the conditions of its own emergence; obviously, the original conditions in which systematic ideas are validated and empirical ones applied are not, and do not resemble, the later conditions of their biography. A cursory glance at the short history of psychoanalysis reveals, moreover, that conduct of psychological therapy in scientific discussion generates more heated controversy than profound enlightenment. Even if this were not the case, psychoanalysis of the existentialist personality would still have to be left to those who work intensively with avowed existentialists. In this sort of inquiry, how-

ever, the existentialist's intentions would probably be misinterpreted and his practical efforts distorted; but if he, too, abandons
his absurd psychology just long enough to make these observations, he modifies his approach because he asserts, by this act, that
processes other than those of immediacy now and then do have
priority.

No structure of psychoanalytic therapy can commit itself to an
absolute and exhaustive theory of its encounter with individual
patients, and still remain free to explore their active processes of
experience. Approaches as different from each other as those of
classical and existentialist analysis involved similar obstacles to
their respective quests for certain and absolute knowledge: classical analysts of the id projected a universal metapsychology to
embrace all human experience, but failed to realize a workable
therapeutic procedure; existentialist analysts, after substituting
abstract expectations from experienced qualities, were burdened
with a metaphysical structure that lacks roots in the ongoing
therapeutic process to be directed and explained. Character
analysts, ego psychologists and interpersonal therapists, on the
other hand, worked successfully with irrational processes that
break loose from unconscious moorings to occupy the foreground
of therapeutic experience, because they never undermined the
structure and function of reflective intelligence, especially during
a patient's attempt to discover and to create a sense of order in
his psychic domain. In fact, they were able to foster this enlargement of awareness just because they respected conscious powers
of intelligence to reconstruct and to reorder the direction of his
previously irrational experience. But they also believed that psychoanalysis, whatever else its meaning or usefulness, is primarily a
science.

Selected Bibliography

F. Alexander *et al.*, *Psychoanalytic Therapy*. New York: Ronald, 1946.

B. Apfelbaum, *Dimensions of Transference in Psychotherapy*. Berkeley & Los Angeles: University of California Press, 1958.

A. Balint and M. Balint, "On Transference and Countertransference," *International Journal of Psychoanalysis*, XX (1939), pp. 223–230.

T. Barber, "Physiological Effects of 'Hypnosis,' " *Psychological Bulletin*, LVIII (1961), pp. 390–419.

J. Breuer and S. Freud, *Studies in Hysteria*. New York: Nervous and Mental Disease Monographs, 1936.

T. Burrow, "The Problem of Transference," *British Journal of Medical Psychology*, VII (1927), pp. 193–202.

M. Cohen, "Countertransference and Anxiety," *Psychiatry*, XV (1952), pp. 231–243.

R. Crowley, "Human Reactions of Analysts to Patients," *Samiksa*, VI (1952), pp. 212–219.

O. Fenichel, *The Psychoanalytic Theory of Neurosis*. New York: Norton, 1945.

S. Ferenczi, *Sex in Psychoanalysis*. New York: Basic Books, 1950.

——, *Theory and Technique of Psychoanalysis*. London: Hogarth Press, 1926.

A. Freud, *The Ego and the Mechanisms of Defence*. New York: International Universities Press, 1946.

S. Freud, *Collected Papers*. Five Volumes. London: Hogarth Press, 1924–1950.

——, *A General Introduction to Psychoanalysis*. Garden City: Garden City, 1943.

——, *New Introductory Lectures on Psychoanalysis*. London: Hogarth Press, 1933.

——, *An Outline of Psychoanalysis*. New York: Norton, 1949.

——, *The Problem of Anxiety*. New York: Norton, 1936.

E. Fromm, *Escape from Freedom*. New York: Rinehart, 1941.

F. Fromm-Reichmann, *Principles of Intensive Psychotherapy*. Chicago: University of Chicago Press, 1950.

P. Greenacre, "The Role of Transference: Practical Considerations in Relation to Psychoanalytic Therapy," *Journal of the American Psychoanalytic Association*, II (1954), pp. 671–684.

R. Grinker, *et al.*, *Psychiatric Social Work*. New York: Basic Books, 1961.

H. Hartmann, "Technical Implications of Ego Psychology," *Psychoanalytic Quarterly*, XX (1951), pp. 31–43.

P. Heimann, "On Countertransference," *International Journal of Psychoanalysis*, XXXI (1950), pp. 81–84.

K. Horney, *New Ways in Psychoanalysis*. New York: Norton, 1939.

E. Kris, "Ego Psychology and Interpretation in Psychoanalytic Therapy," *Psychoanalytic Quarterly*, XX (1951), pp. 15–30.

D. Lagache, "Le Probleme du Transfert," *Revue Française de Psychoanalyse*, XVI (1952), pp. 5–115.

——, "The Problem of Transference," in J. Frosch *et al.*, *Annual Survey of Psychoanalysis*. New York: International Universities Press, 1952.

E. Levenson, "Changing Time Concepts in Psychoanalysis," *American Journal of Psychotherapy*, XII (1958), pp. 64–78.

M. Little, "Countertransference and the Patient's Response to It," *International Journal of Psychoanalysis*, XXXII (1951), pp. 320–340.

I. Macalpine, "The Development of the Transference," *Psychoanalytic Quarterly* XIX (1950), pp. 501–539.

K. Menninger, *Theory of Psychoanalytic Technique*. New York: Basic Books, 1958.

J. Meerloo and M. Coleman, "The Transference Function: A Study of Normal and Pathological Transference," *Psychoanalytic Review*, XXXVIII (1951), pp. 205–221.

H. Nunberg, "Transference and Reality," *International Journal of Psychoanalysis*, XXXII (1951), pp. 1–9.

D. Orr, "Transference and Countertransference: a Historical Survey," *Journal of the American Psychoanalytic Association*, II (1954), pp. 621–670.

S. Rado, "Recent Advances in Psychoanalytic Therapy," in *Proceedings of the Association for Research in Nervous and Mental Disease*. Baltimore: Williams & Wilkins, 1953.

O. Rank and S. Ferenczi, *The Development of Psychoanalysis*. New York: Nervous and Mental Disease Monographs, 1925.

D. Rapaport, "The Structure of Psychoanalytic Theory," *Psychological Issues*, II (1960), pp. 1–158.

W. Reich, *Character Analysis*. New York: Orgone Institute Press, 1945.

J. Rioch, "The Transference Phenomenon in Psychoanalytic Therapy," *Psychiatry*, VI (1943), pp. 147–156.

J. Rosen, "Transference: A Concept of Its Origin, Its Purpose and Its Fate," *Acta Psychotherapeutica, Psychosomatica et Orthopaedagogica*, II (1954), pp. 300–314.

E. Schachtel, *Metamorphosis*. New York: Basic Books, 1959.

R. Schonbar, "Transference as a Bridge to the Future," *American Journal of Psychotherapy*, XVII (1963), pp. 286–298.

W. Silverberg, "The Concept of Transference," *Psychoanalytic Quarterly*, XVII (1948), pp. 303–321.

R. Sobel, "Role Conflict or Resistance," *American Journal of Psychotherapy*, XVIII (1964), pp. 25–34.

J. Spiegel, "The Social Roles of Doctor and Patient in Psychoanalysis and Psychotherapy," *Psychiatry*, XVII (1954), pp. 369–376.

J. Strachey, "The Nature of the Therapeutic Action of Psychoanalysis," *International Journal of Psychoanalysis*, XV (1934), pp. 127–159.

H. Sullivan, *Conceptions of Modern Psychiatry*. Washington: W. A. White Psychiatric Foundation, 1947.

——, *The Interpersonal Theory of Psychiatry*. New York: Norton, 1953.

E. Tauber, "Observations on Counter-Transference, *Samiksa*, VI (1952), pp. 220–228.

E. Tauber and M. Green, *Prelogical Experience*. New York: Basic Books, 1959.

C. Thompson, "Counter-Transference," *Samiksa*, VI (1952), pp. 205–211.

——, "Development of Awareness of Transference in a Markedly Detached Personality," *International Journal of Psychoanalysis*, XIX (1938), pp. 199–209.

——, *Psychoanalysis*. New York: Hermitage House, 1950.

——, "The Role of the Analyst's Personality in Therapy," *American Journal of Psychotherapy*, X (1956), pp. 347–359.

——, "Transference and Character Analysis," *Samiksa*, VII (1953), pp. 260–270.

L. Tower, "Countertransference," *Journal of the American Psychoanalytic Association*, IV (1956), pp. 224–255.

S. Tower, "Management of Paranoid Trends in Treatment of a Post-Psychotic Obsessional Condition," *Psychiatry*, X (1947), pp. 137–141.

M. White, "Sullivan and Treatment," in P. Mullahy (ed.), *The Contributions of Harry Stack Sullivan*. New York: Hermitage House, 1952.

L. Wolberg, *Medical Hypnosis*. Two Volumes. New York: Grune & Stratton, 1948.

B. Wolstein, *Countertransference*. New York: Grune & Stratton, 1959.

——, *Freedom to Experience*. New York: Grune & Stratton, 1964.

Index